Contents

Generous Coconut Orange Creamsicles!

Conclusion

Introduction

Since you have this book in your hand, I am assuming that you have decided to jump into the wonderful world of Ketogenic Diet!

I am happy to tell you, that you have come to the right place!

I have carefully designed this book to contain extremely delicious and easy to make recipes Ketogenic Recipes, alongside a very beefy introductory chapter that covers most of the fundamentals of a Ketogenic Diet.

Since I have written this chapter in a very easy to understand way, you will be able to jump into a Keto diet even if you are an amateur!

So, let us start with the basics first.

The exact definition of a Ketogenic Diet

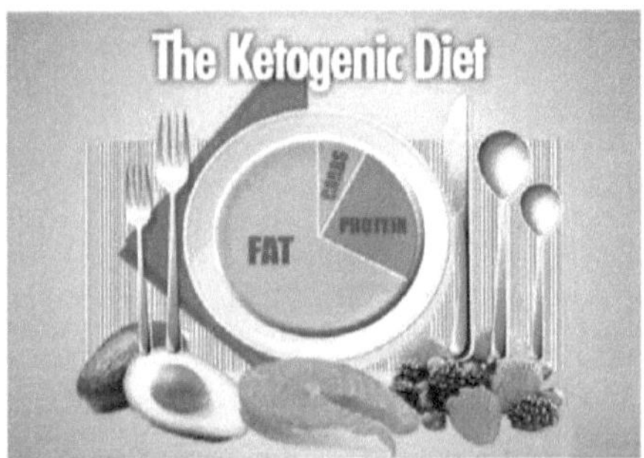

When talking about a Ketogenic diet, the very first thing that you should understand is the definition of the word "Keto."

This is a word that is derived from a human metabolic process known as "Ketosis," which is a process that helps the body to produce a chemical called "Ketones."

The main objective of a Keto diet is to generally lower down the intake of Carbohydrates in your body. This is the reason why a Ketogenic diet is also known as Low-Carb Diet or even a High-Protein Diet.

Throughout the rest of the chapter, I will be referring to it as simply Ketogenic Diet

The basic working procedure of a Ketogenic Diet

To understand the process through which a Ketogenic Diet work, you must first appreciate the fact that whenever our body is exposed to a large amount of Carbohydrate, the body tends to increase its production of Glucose and Insulin and release them into the blood steam.

Glucose is possibly the most easily convertible molecule that is present in your body. Whenever you are under stress and/or your body is doing something heavy, it starts to convert glucose to get the energy required for your body to work properly.

The Insulin on the other hand helps to maintain the level of Glucose in our bloodstream. Whenever the level of Glucose gets incredibly high, the production of insulin is increased which lowers down the Glucose to minimal safe levels.

Here's the thing now. Whenever glucose is present in abundance in your body, it also greatly decreases the level of fat that is burned via hard work, since the body burns the excess glucose in order the get its energy.

This is also one of the reasons why you might not be obtaining satisfactory results even after hours upon hours of crucial workout sessions!

Whenever the amount of Carbohydrate present in our body starts to go down, it enters into a phase known as "Ketosis" which is basically the body's natural response mechanism which allows it to tackle the body deal with a lower food intake.

In this phase, the body produces a larger number of Ketones which breaks down more fat from the body instead of Carbohydrates/glucose to produce the required energy.

Understanding the basics of Ketosis

As mentioned in the previous section, the main objective of a Ketogenic Diet is to encourage the internal mechanism of your body to enter into a state of Ketosis.

Essentially what happens here is that, whenever you are depriving your body of Carbohydrates, it starts to burn down fat for energy due to the shortage of Carbohydrates. During this process, a chemical called "Ketones."

Ketone is essentially the chemical which encourages the body to break down fat instead of glucose and supply energy to the body.

How to understand that your body is in Ketosis

Since you now have the idea of the basic concept of Ketosis, it is essential for your to understand the basic signs and symptoms of Ketosis. Once you have started your Keto diet, should you experience any of these symptoms, then rest assured that you have entered Ketosis.

- Your mouth will feel dry, and you feel have increased thirst
- The number of washroom visits will increase as you might need to urinate more often.
- Your breath will have a slight "Fruity" smell to it that will resemble that of a nail polish
- Aside from those three, you will obviously get the sensation mentioned above of having a low hunger level and increased bodily energy.

Tips to enter optimal levels of Ketosis

By now you should be clear that the effectiveness of a Ketogenic diet depend on the level of your Ketosis your body is able to achieve.

While simply lowering your carbohydrate intake will most definitely help you enter Ketosis, the following tips will not only help you to enhance the effectiveness of your Ketosis, but also allow your body to stay in a state of Ketosis for a longer period of time.

- Keep your daily carbohydrate intake below 20 carbs
- Keep your protein levels at around 70g per day
- Don't starve! Swallow adequate level of fat. Remember that the body is going to need fat to burn fat.

- Try to avoid snack times and stick to your breakfast, lunch and dinner meals with nothing in between.

Some physical effects to keep in mind

Going through such a drastic change in your diet, your body is bound to experience some physical changes due to the changes in your overall homeostatic functions.

Eventually, the body will start to habituate itself to the type of your meals that you are taking in by producing more enzymes to digest those particular types of meals easily.

During the early stage of your diet, some minor side effects that you might experience include:

- Dizziness
- Aggravation
- Headaches
- Keto-Flu
- Mental Fogginess

Aside from those, some symptoms which you should be aware of are:

- **Frequent desire to urinate:** Since Ketosis will cause your body to burn up more fat, the glycogen gets stored up. In this situation, your Kidneys will start to process a lot of water and excrete them, increasing your desire to urinate.
- **Hypoglycemia:** This simply means that your sugar level might lower down
- **Constipation:** This is yet another side effect experience by some which take place due to dehydration and lower salt presence in the body. But this can very easily be tackled by drinking more water
- **Increased Sugar Craving:** During the early stage of your diet, you might get a serious craving for sugar. To tackle this, simply take some extra protein and Vitamin B Complex. A good and healthy walk works good as well.
- **Diarrhea:** This is a common issue which is faced by some people during the first few days, but it resolves itself automatically after a few days.

- **Sleep problem:** This might be a result of the reduced levels of serotonin or insulin.

When the body is in a state of Ketosis, it causes plenty of electrolytes to be flushed out from the body which is the main reason for such effects of taking place. This diuretic effect can be tackled by increasing the level of water consumption during a Ketogenic Diet. Another advice would be to increase your normal salt intake which will also help to rejuvenate the levels of electrolytes.

So, keep in mind that if you are experiencing any of the above-mentioned symptoms, they are pretty normal and there is nothing to be worried about!

Understanding the concept of body weight and BMI

Let's face it; the main reason for you exploring the concepts of Ketogenic diet is to find how it can help you trim down your body weight!

But have you ever wondered when we are talking about "Weight," what exactly are we referring to?

Well, in Layman's term we are talking about the mass of our body, incidentally, the bulk of the mass comes from the amount of water, bones, body fat and muscle present in our body.

In short, everything that makes up the whole skeletal infrastructure comprises our mass.

Following that definition, when a person is referred to as being either "Fat" or even "Obese," they are being said that they have a significant amount of body fat or "mass" that is hampering their overall body physique and health.

Professionals such as Doctors or Nurses, though, often follow something which is called the BMI or Body Mass Index to assess the condition of their physique.

For those of you who are getting to know of BMI for the first time, BMI is basically a method of measurement that is done by comparing the weight and height of an individual. The values are used in conjunction with the given formula below to get a BMI. The BMI value is then crosschecked with a BMI table similar to the one given below to properly assess the physique of someone.

$$\text{Body Mass Index} = \frac{\text{Weight (in kg)}}{\text{Height}^2 \text{ (in m)}}$$

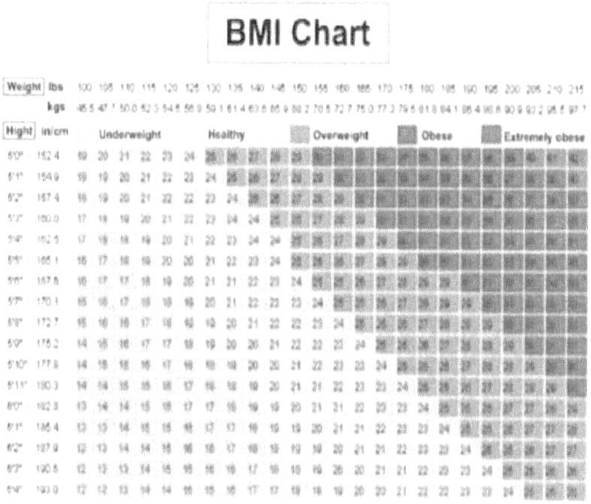

BMI Chart

Weight	lbs	100	105	110	115	120	125	130	135	140	145	150	155	160	165	170	175	180	185	190	195	200	205	210	215
	kgs	45.5	47.7	50.0	52.3	54.5	56.9	59.1	61.4	63.6	65.9	68.2	70.5	72.7	75.0	77.3	79.5	81.8	84.1	86.4	88.6	90.9	93.2	95.5	97.7

Legend: Underweight — Healthy — Overweight — Obese — Extremely obese

Hight	in/cm																								
5'0"	152.4	19	20	21	22	23	24	[illegible]	[illegible]	[illegible]	[illegible]	[illegible]	[illegible]	[illegible]	[illegible]	[illegible]	[illegible]	[illegible]	[illegible]	[illegible]	[illegible]	[illegible]	[illegible]	[illegible]	[illegible]
5'1"	154.9	19	19	20	21	22	23	24	[illegible]	[illegible]	[illegible]	[illegible]	[illegible]	[illegible]	[illegible]	[illegible]	[illegible]	[illegible]	[illegible]	[illegible]	[illegible]	[illegible]	[illegible]	[illegible]	[illegible]
5'2"	157.4	18	19	20	21	22	22	23	24	[illegible]	[illegible]	[illegible]	[illegible]	[illegible]	[illegible]	[illegible]	[illegible]	[illegible]	[illegible]	[illegible]	[illegible]	[illegible]	[illegible]	[illegible]	[illegible]
5'3"	160.0	17	18	19	20	21	22	23	24	24	[illegible]	[illegible]	[illegible]	[illegible]	[illegible]	[illegible]	[illegible]	[illegible]	[illegible]	[illegible]	[illegible]	[illegible]	[illegible]	[illegible]	[illegible]
5'4"	162.5	17	18	18	19	20	21	22	23	24	24	[illegible]	[illegible]	[illegible]	[illegible]	[illegible]	[illegible]	[illegible]	[illegible]	[illegible]	[illegible]	[illegible]	[illegible]	[illegible]	[illegible]
5'5"	165.1	16	17	18	19	20	20	21	22	23	24	[illegible]	[illegible]	[illegible]	[illegible]	[illegible]	[illegible]	[illegible]	[illegible]	[illegible]	[illegible]	[illegible]	[illegible]	[illegible]	[illegible]
5'6"	167.6	16	17	17	18	19	20	21	21	22	23	24	[illegible]	[illegible]	[illegible]	[illegible]	[illegible]	[illegible]	[illegible]	[illegible]	[illegible]	[illegible]	[illegible]	[illegible]	[illegible]
5'7"	170.1	15	16	17	18	19	19	20	21	22	23	23	24	[illegible]	[illegible]	[illegible]	[illegible]	[illegible]	[illegible]	[illegible]	[illegible]	[illegible]	[illegible]	[illegible]	[illegible]
5'8"	172.7	15	16	16	17	18	19	19	20	21	22	22	23	24	[illegible]	[illegible]	[illegible]	[illegible]	[illegible]	[illegible]	[illegible]	[illegible]	[illegible]	[illegible]	[illegible]
5'9"	175.2	14	15	16	17	17	18	19	20	20	21	22	22	23	24	[illegible]	[illegible]	[illegible]	[illegible]	[illegible]	[illegible]	[illegible]	[illegible]	[illegible]	[illegible]
5'10"	177.8	14	15	16	16	17	18	18	19	20	20	21	22	23	23	24	[illegible]	[illegible]	[illegible]	[illegible]	[illegible]	[illegible]	[illegible]	[illegible]	[illegible]
5'11"	180.3	14	14	15	16	16	17	18	18	19	20	21	21	22	23	23	24	[illegible]	[illegible]	[illegible]	[illegible]	[illegible]	[illegible]	[illegible]	[illegible]
6'0"	182.8	13	14	14	15	16	17	17	18	19	19	20	21	21	22	23	23	24	[illegible]	[illegible]	[illegible]	[illegible]	[illegible]	[illegible]	[illegible]
6'1"	185.4	13	13	14	15	15	16	17	17	18	19	19	20	21	21	22	23	23	24	[illegible]	[illegible]	[illegible]	[illegible]	[illegible]	[illegible]
6'2"	187.9	12	13	14	14	15	16	16	17	18	18	19	19	20	21	21	22	23	23	24	[illegible]	[illegible]	[illegible]	[illegible]	[illegible]
6'3"	190.5	12	13	13	14	15	15	16	16	17	18	18	19	20	20	21	21	22	23	23	24	[illegible]	[illegible]	[illegible]	[illegible]
6'4"	193.0	12	12	13	14	14	15	15	16	17	17	18	18	19	20	20	21	22	22	23	23	24	[illegible]	[illegible]	[illegible]

The standards you see in the graph were set by an extensive research done by the World Health Organization, so they are extremely accurate. So, imagine that you have a body index of 25-30, it would make you overweight. Alternatively, if you have an index of 30+, you would be obese.

Sadly, though, at the time of writing, the level of people suffering from obesity and a high body fat percentage was at an all-time high. In fact, in 2014 it was estimated that almost 600 million adults were suffering from obesity while 42 million of the total obese population were children under five! Thank you excellent fast foods!

Scientific evidence supporting the power of Ketogenic Diet

You have already seen that a Ketogenic diet makes some pretty big claims when it comes to trimming down body weight.

Now, I definitely don't want you to believe in word of mouth! In fact, the following is a look at a very in-depth study that was conducted recently.

A team of around eight research scientists took a notion of bringing into contrast the effectiveness of an Atkins Diet (equivalent to a Keto Diet) with three other different forms of diet over a period of 12 months completely randomized control trial.

The participants of this experiment included a broad range of 311 individuals who ranged from obese people and women who had menopause. It was strictly maintained though that none of the patients had a history of any form of cardiovascular or diabetic symptoms.

An average age of 41 years was measured of the sample, following a BMI of 32 with body fat which clocked at a percentage of 40%

After establishing these basal standards, the scientists divide the whole sample into four different groups based on the type of diet they were exposed to.

- Group-1 comprised of 76 people were instructed to consume an Ornish Diet which had just about 10% lowered down calorie in comparison to the fatty foods.
- Group 2 had 79 participants and they were asked to go through a LEARN Diet which comprised of the same 10% fewer calories, but this time it came from the saturated fats, while 55-60% of the calorie came from the carbohydrates. The psychological and physiological activities of this group were also monitored.
- Group 3 comprising of 79 people was exposed to something called the "Zone Diet" which consisting of roughly 30%, 40% and 30% distribution of calories coming from protein, carbohydrate and fats respectively.
- Group 4 had a number of 77 participants. They were treated with a diet of the low-carb "Atkins" diet.

For all of the diets, each subject was exposed to only 20 grams of carbs per day for 2-3 months. After which they were instructed to eat 50g per day for the coming 9-10 months.

The test subjects were strictly asked to maintain the specified calorie deficit and take professional support to adjust their level of diet accordingly to ensure that they are able to adhere to the specified diet while being healthy as well.

Aside from the diet routine, the researchers also invoked a nice routine of exercise and nutritional supplements to make sure that they were not losing their healthy physique.

As you can already tell by now, the whole experiment was pretty elaborate and well thought out and the conclusion, well unsurprisingly all of the diets had shown a good amount of reduction in BMI and overall weight alongside body fat percentage. But, the one that showed the greatest decline was the Atkins diet which closely resembled the diet of a Ketogenic style.

The graph up pretty much sums up the whole scenario nicely. As you can see, the decrease in BMI of the Atkins group decreases by 1.65. In comparison, it only fell by 0.92 in the LEARN group, 0.77 in the Ornish group and a disappointing 0.53 in the Zone group.

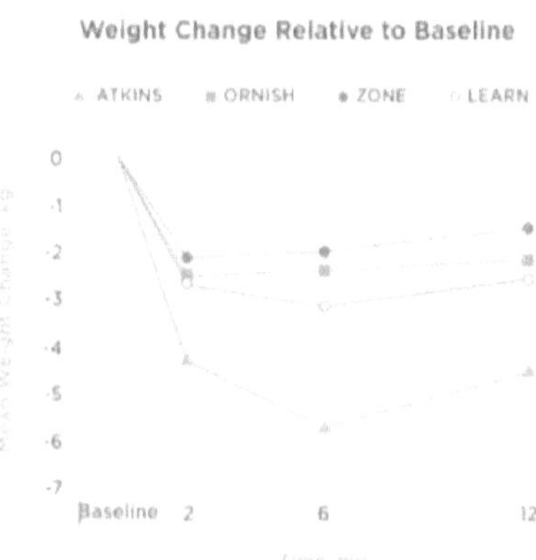

The same is seen in the bar chart below.

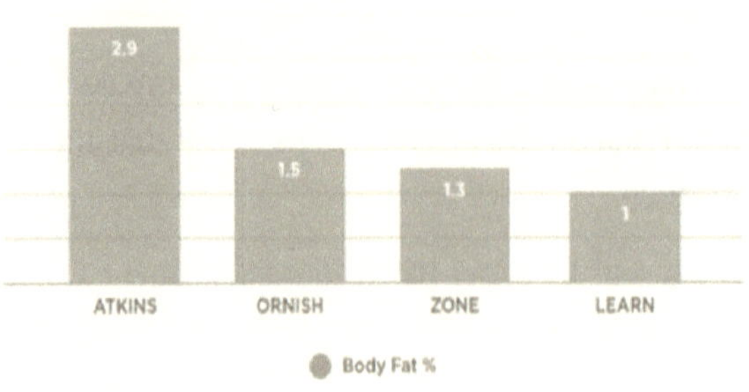

Credit: Taken from www.ruled.me

But not that's not all! If you just have a look at the decline in body fat percentage that was trimmed down, the effects were more astonishing! The recorded rate decrease from the Atkins diet was at an astounding 2.9% while the others had a decline of around 1.5%, 1.3% and 1% in the Ornish, Zone, and LEARN group respectively. This even further supports the theory of the effectiveness of a low carb diet.

So, the conclusion? Yes. Through the tests done under an Atkins Diet, it can very easily be inferred that a Ketogenic Diet has the potentiality to trim down those pesky body fats and return you to the physique which you were dreaming for!

This incidentally meant that the Atkins group, which was on a diet with much decrease carb intake that the other two groups showed significantly plausible results.

Consequently, this led to people all around the world to believe that it is indeed possible to trim down fat using a diet of Low-Carb, which is in our case, A Ketogenic Diet.

Advantages of Ketogenic Diet

So, about I let you know a bit about the different advantages and benefits of going into a Ketogenic Diet!

✓	A good Keto diet will help you to lower the levels of bad cholesterol so to prevent arterial blocks from occurring

✓	Energy taken from burning body fat will always keep you energetic since body fat is present in abundance in our body

✓	The levels of LDL will decrease which will make the body less prone to suffer from Type-2 Diabetes

✓	You won't always feel hungry

✓	Ketosis helps to improve skin condition and prevent acnes or skin inflammation from taking place.

But what about the other benefits of Ketogenic Diet, other than trimming down your weight you ask?

- A Ketogenic diet directly helps to increase the level of fat burnt throughout the whole day through exercise and daily activities
- A Keto Diet will cause the body to consume a significant amount of protein, consequently promoting the weight loss of the body.
- When the body is restricted from consuming Carbohydrates, the calorie intake will also lower down further contributing to weight loss.
- A process called Gluconeogenesis will kick in as well which will cause the body to burn even more fat.
- Speaking of burning fat, A Ketogenic diet will also help you to Suppress your Appetite, so you won't have to go out and eat now and then and bulk up, even more, fat.

The ingredients to be aware of

Fats

Go For

- Saturated Fat like coconut oil ghee
- Monosaturated Fat like olive, macadamia, almond oil
- Polyunsaturated Omega 3s as sardines
- Medium Chain Triglycerides such as fatty acid

- Lard
- Chicken Fat
- Duck Fat
- Goose Fat

Not Go For

- Refined Fats and Oil as sunflower, soybean, corn oil, etc.
- Trans Fat such as margarine

Protein

Go For

- Grass fed meat
- Harvested seafood and wild caught meat
- Free-range organic egg
- Beef
- Lamb
- Goat
- Venison
- Pastured Pork
- Poultry

Not Go For

- Factory packed animal foods and produced

Vegetable

Go For

- Leafy green vegetables
- Low carb vegetables
- Swiss chard
- Bok Choy
- Lettuce
- Chard
- Chives
- Endives

* Radicchio

Not Go For

* High starchy= high carb vegetables such as peas, potatoes, yucca, beans, legumes.

Dairy Products

Go For

* Dairy products such as yogurt, sour cream, cottage cheese, goat cheese

Not Go For

* Milk

Fruits

Go For

* In general, go for fruits that are on low carb and have more fat such as berries, avocados, etc.

Not Go For

* Try to avoid dried fruits that are high in sugar content

Drinks

Go For

* Water
* Black Coffee
* Unsweetened and Herbal Teas
* Nut Milks
* Light Beet
* Wine

Not Go For

- Drinks such as Pepsi or Coke
- High Fructose Syrup
- Nectar
- Honey
- Sodas

Sweets

Go For

- Stevia
- Xylitol
- Erythritol
- Inulin
- Monk Fruit Powder
- Cocoa Dark Chocolate

Not Go For

- Milk

Tips for a healthy Keto journey

- Get yourself a carb counter to keep your daily carb intake in check.
- Make sure to get rid of all of your high-carb produces from the cupboard.
- Try to prepare a good meal plan (a demo is provided in this book).
- Slowly try to alter your daily habits and accept new ones to make sure that they would complement your new diet style
- Try to stay as much hydrated as you can by drinking water.
- Always make sure to keep your sodium intake in check. It will make your Keto journey much more pleasant. Some tips may include.

  - ✓ Drinking organic broth if possible
  - ✓ Taking a just a pinch of pink salt with you consumed meals
  - ✓ Adding about ¼ teaspoon of pink salt to 16 ounces of water

consumed

✓ Adding vegetables such as kelp to your dishes

✓ Eating up vegetables such as cucumber or celery for a more natural approach to sodium replenishment

- Try to include a basic amount of physical exercise into your diet regime as well. It would not only make you healthy but also accelerate the effectiveness of your Keto diet. A general exercise routine may include

  - ❖ Monday: Resistance training for upper body (20 minutes)
  - ❖ Tuesday: Resistance training for Lower Body (20 minutes)
  - ❖ Wednesday: Long walk of 30 minutes
  - ❖ Thursday: Resistance training for upper body (20 minutes)
  - ❖ Friday: Resistance training for Lower Body (20 minutes)
  - ❖ Sat/Sun: Recreational time.

A perfect 7 days meal plan

The amount of Carb that you are allowed to take while on a Ketogenic diet largely depends on the amount of fat you want to lose and how quickly you want to do it.

The ideal limit lies somewhere around 20-100g of carbs per day. For our meal plan, I will be keeping the carbs under 100g.

Keep in mind that you will be able to modify the meal plan and extend it as well accordingly, using the recipes provided in this book.

Day 1	**Total Count:** • Protein: 79 • Carbs: 21g • Fats: 155g • Calories: 1823
Breakfast	**Intense Flatbread With Apple Flavors** • Protein: 16g • Carbs: 5g • Fats: 20g

	• Calories: 255
Snack	**Time Pass White Pizza Frittata** • Calories: 298 • Fat: 23g • Carbohydrates: 2.9g • Protein: 19g
Lunch	**Braised Beef Bone Short Ribs** • Calories: 550 • Fat: 39g • Carbohydrates: 4g • Protein: 14g
Dinner	**Walnut Crusted Salmon** • Protein: 20g • Carbs: 4g • Fats: 43g • Calories: 373
Desert	**Miniature Vanilla Cloud Muffins** • Protein: 10g • Carbs: 5g • Fats: 30g • Calories: 347

Day 2	**Total Count:** • Protein: 65 • Carbs: 33g • Fats: 96g • Calories: 1296
Breakfast	**A Good Morning Brownie Muffin** • Calories: 183 • Fat: 13g • Carbohydrates: 9g • Protein: 7g
	Cute Miniature Spiced Muffins • Calories: 42

Snack	<ul><li>Fat: 2.9g</li><li>Carbohydrates: 1.23g</li><li>Protein: 1.84g</li></ul>
Lunch	**Crazy Homemade Bolognese**<ul><li>Calories: 237</li><li>Fat: 14g</li><li>Carbohydrates: 14g</li><li>Protein: 16g</li></ul>
Dinner	**The Original Keto Sushi**<ul><li>Calories: 353</li><li>Fat: 25</li><li>Carbohydrates: 5.7</li><li>Protein: 18</li></ul>
Desert	**The Greatest McGriddle Casserole**<ul><li>Protein: 22.6g</li><li>Carbs: 2.9g</li><li>Fats: 41g</li><li>Calories: 481</li></ul>

Day 3	**Total Count:**<ul><li>Protein: 69</li><li>Carbs: 22g</li><li>Fats: 111g</li><li>Calories: 1366</li></ul>
Breakfast	**Fabulous Poached Eggs With Tomatoes**<ul><li>Protein: 16g</li><li>Carbs: 5g</li><li>Fats: 20g</li><li>Calories: 255</li></ul>
Snack	**Delicious Stuffed Peppers**<ul><li>Calories: 313</li><li>Fat: 24g</li><li>Carbohydrates: 9g</li></ul>

	• Protein: 15g
Lunch	**Super Cool Nasi Lemak** • Protein: 1.4g • Carbs: 0.7g • Fats: 2.7g • Calories: 32
Dinner	**A Chicken Sandwich Filled With Bacon and Avocado** • Protein: 22g • Carbs: 4g • Fats: 28g • Calories: 361
Desert	**Soft Caprese Salad** • Protein: 15g • Carbs: 3.5g • Fats: 36g • Calories: 405

Day 4	**Total Count:** • Protein: 79 • Carbs: 21g • Fats: 155g • Calories: 1823
Breakfast	**Intense Flatbread With Apple Flavors** • Protein: 16g • Carbs: 5g • Fats: 20g • Calories: 255
Snack	**Time Pass White Pizza Frittata** • Calories: 298 • Fat: 23g • Carbohydrates: 2.9g • Protein: 19g
	Braised Beef Bone Short Ribs

Lunch	<ul><li>Calories: 550</li><li>Fat: 39g</li><li>Carbohydrates: 4g</li><li>Protein: 14g</li></ul>
Dinner	**Walnut Crusted Salmon**<ul><li>Protein: 20g</li><li>Carbs: 4g</li><li>Fats: 43g</li><li>Calories: 373</li></ul>
Desert	**Miniature Vanilla Cloud Muffins**<ul><li>Protein: 10g</li><li>Carbs: 5g</li><li>Fats: 30g</li><li>Calories: 347</li></ul>

Day 5	**Total Count:**<ul><li>Protein: 65</li><li>Carbs: 33g</li><li>Fats: 96g</li><li>Calories: 1296</li></ul>
Breakfast	**A Good Morning Brownie Muffin**<ul><li>Calories: 183</li><li>Fat: 13g</li><li>Carbohydrates: 9g</li><li>Protein: 7g</li></ul>
Snack	**Cute Miniature Spiced Muffins**<ul><li>Calories: 42</li><li>Fat: 2.9g</li><li>Carbohydrates: 1.23g</li><li>Protein: 1.84g</li></ul>
Lunch	**Crazy Homemade Bolognese**<ul><li>Calories: 237</li><li>Fat: 14g</li><li>Carbohydrates: 14g</li><li>Protein: 16g</li></ul>

Dinner	**The Original Keto Sushi** • Calories: 353 • Fat: 25 • Carbohydrates: 5.7 • Protein: 18
Desert	**The Greatest McGriddle Casserole** • Protein: 22.6g • Carbs: 2.9g • Fats: 41g • Calories: 481

Day 6	**Total Count:** • Protein: 69 • Carbs: 22g • Fats: 111g • Calories: 1366
Breakfast	**Fabulous Poached Eggs With Tomatoes** • Protein: 16g • Carbs: 5g • Fats: 20g • Calories: 255
Snack	**Delicious Stuffed Peppers** • Calories: 313 • Fat: 24g • Carbohydrates: 9g • Protein: 15g
Lunch	**Super Cool Nasi Lemak** • Protein: 1.4g • Carbs: 0.7g • Fats: 2.7g • Calories: 32
	A Chicken Sandwich Filled With Bacon and Avocado

Dinner	<ul><li>Protein: 22g</li><li>Carbs: 4g</li><li>Fats: 28g</li><li>Calories: 361</li></ul>
Desert	**Soft Caprese Salad**<ul><li>Protein: 15g</li><li>Carbs: 3.5g</li><li>Fats: 36g</li><li>Calories: 405</li></ul>

Day 7	**Total Count:**<ul><li>Protein: 65</li><li>Carbs: 33g</li><li>Fats: 96g</li><li>Calories: 1296</li></ul>
Breakfast	**A Good Morning Brownie Muffin**<ul><li>Calories: 183</li><li>Fat: 13g</li><li>Carbohydrates: 9g</li><li>Protein: 7g</li></ul>
Snack	**Cute Miniature Spiced Muffins**<ul><li>Calories: 42</li><li>Fat: 2.9g</li><li>Carbohydrates: 1.23g</li><li>Protein: 1.84g</li></ul>
Lunch	**Crazy Homemade Bolognese**<ul><li>Calories: 237</li><li>Fat: 14g</li><li>Carbohydrates: 14g</li><li>Protein: 16g</li></ul>
Dinner	**The Original Keto Sushi**<ul><li>Calories: 353</li><li>Fat: 25</li><li>Carbohydrates: 5.7</li></ul>

	• Protein: 18
Desert	**The Greatest McGriddle Casserole** • Protein: 22.6g • Carbs: 2.9g • Fats: 41g • Calories: 481

Chapter 1: Breakfast Recipes

Intense Flatbread With Apple Flavors

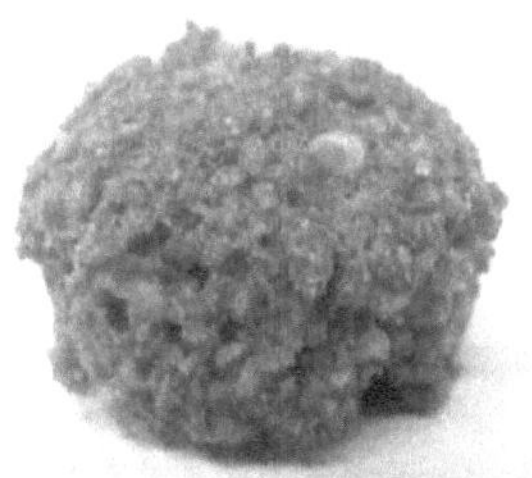

Serving: 8

Prep Time: 15 minutes

Cook Time: 20 minutes

<u>Ingredients</u>

Ingredients required for the crust

- 2 cups of grated partially skimmed mozzarella cheese
- ¾ cup of almond flour
- 2 tablespoon of sea salt
- 1/8 teaspoon of dried thyme

Ingredients needed for the topping

- 2 cup of grated Mexican cheese
- ½ of a small onion sliced into thin portions
- ¼ of a medium sized apple. Seeded and cored with the skin intact
- 4 ounce of low carb ham sliced into chunks
- 1/8 teaspoon of dried thyme
- Salt as required
- Pepper as required

<u>How To</u>

1. The first step is to preheat your oven to a temperature of 425 degrees Fahrenheit

2. Next, two about two pieces of parchment paper which should be about 2 inches large than a 12-inch pan pizza

3. Prepare a nice double boiler

4. Take a sauce pot and fill it up with just enough water and bring the water to simmer. Once brought to simmer, low down the heat

5. Take the mixing bowl prepared for the double boiler and toss in the cream cheese, mozzarella cheese, almond flour, salt and thyme

6. Gently place the bowl over the simmering pot and keep stirring it continuously while being careful of the steam

7. Once the cheese have melted down and ingredients are combined, pour down the mixture to one of the previously prepared parchment paper and knead it for a few minutes

8. Roll up the whole dough into a ball and place it on the center of the paper

9. Gently keep patting it until a nice circular shape has appeared

10. Cover it with the other parchment paper.

11. Take a rolling pin and keep rolling the dough until it has a nice 12-inch radius

12. Place the prepared dough on a pizza pan and take a fork to drill holes all over

13. Bake it for about 8 minutes

14. Once a golden texture has appeared, lower down the heat to 350 degrees Fahrenheit

15. Sprinkle about ¼ cup of the cheese

16. Finely place the sliced onion, apple and ham

17. Bake it again for 5-7 minutes until the cheese has melted and browned

18. Place it on a cooling rack and let it cool for about 3 minutes before cutting into 8 individual slices

<u>Nutrition Values(Per Serving)</u>

- Protein: 16g
- Carbs: 5g
- Fats: 20g
- Calories: 255
- Fiber: 1g

A Good Morning Brownie Muffin

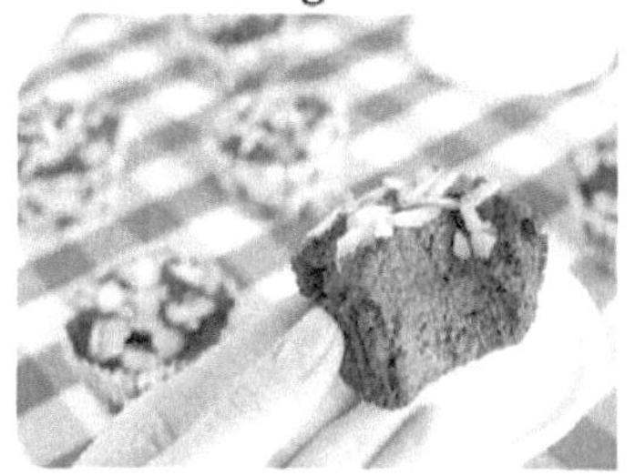

Serving: 5

Prep Time: 10 minutes

Cook Time: 35 minutes

Ingredients

- 1 cup of Golden Flaxseed Meal
- ¼ cup of cocoa powder
- 1 tablespoon of Cinnamon
- ½ tablespoon of Baking Powder
- ½ a teaspoon of Salt
- 1 piece of large egg
- 2 tablespoon of Coconut Oil
- ¼ cup of Sugar-free Caramel Syrup
- ½ a cup of Pumpkin Puree
- 1 teaspoon of Vanilla Extract
- 1 teaspoon of Apple Cider Vinegar
- ¼ cup of Silvered Almond

How To

1. The first step is to prepare your oven and pre-heat it to a temperature of 350 degrees Fahrenheit
2. Take a mixing bowl and toss in all of the ingredients in the bowl and combine everything
3. Take a muff tin and line it up with 6 paper liners
4. Scoop up the fill up the about ¼ of each of muffin liner
5. Sprinkle a bit of almond on top of the batter
6. Put it in your oven and let it bake for about 15 minutes

7. Once done, serve warm

Nutrition

- Calories: 183
- Fat: 13g
- Carbohydrates: 9g
- Protein: 7g

Fabulous Poached Eggs With Tomatoes

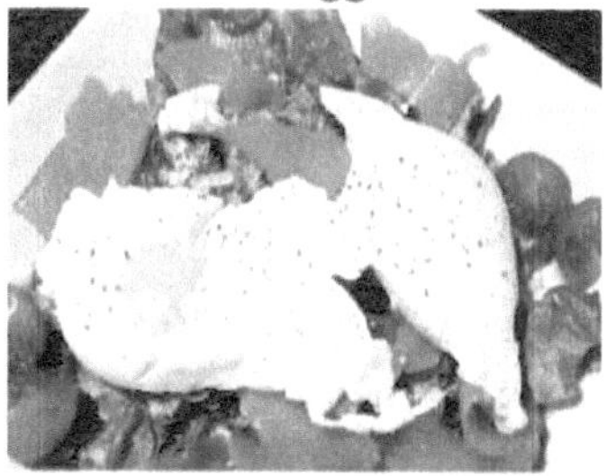

Serving: 4

Prep Time: 5 minutes

Cook Time: 5 minutes

<u>Ingredients</u>

Ingredients required for the crust

- 2 cups of grated partially skimmed mozzarella cheese
- ¾ cup of almond flour
- 2 tablespoon of sea salt
- 1/8 teaspoon of dried thyme

Ingredients needed for the topping

- 2 cup of grated Mexican cheese
- ½ of a small onion sliced into thin portions
- ¼ of a medium sized apple. Seeded and cored with the skin intact
- 4 ounce of low carb ham sliced into chunks
- 1/8 teaspoon of dried thyme
- Salt as required
- Pepper as required

<u>How To</u>

1. The first step is to preheat your oven to a temperature of 425 degrees Fahrenheit

2. Next, two about two pieces of parchment paper which should be about 2 inches large than a 12-inch pan pizza

3. Prepare a nice double boiler

4. Take a sauce pot and fill it up with just enough water and bring the water to simmer. Once brought to simmer, low down the heat

5. Take the mixing bowl prepared for the double boiler and toss in the cream cheese, mozzarella cheese, almond flour, salt and thyme

6. Gently place the bowl over the simmering pot and keep stirring it continuously while being careful of the steam

7. Once the cheese have melted down and ingredients are combined, pour down the mixture to one of the previously prepared parchment paper and knead it for a few minutes

8. Roll up the whole dough into a ball and place it on the center of the paper

9. Gently keep patting it until a nice circular shape has appeared

10. Cover it with the other parchment paper.

11. Take a rolling pin and keep rolling the dough until it has a nice 12-inch radius

12. Place the prepared dough on a pizza pan and take a fork to drill holes all over

13. Bake it for about 8 minutes

14. Once a golden texture has appeared, lower down the heat to 350 degrees Fahrenheit

15. Sprinkle about ¼ cup of the cheese

16. Finely place the sliced onion, apple and ham

17. Bake it again for 5-7 minutes until the cheese has melted and browned

18. Place it on a cooling rack and let it cool for about 3 minutes before cutting into 8 individual slices

<u>Nutrition Values(Per Serving)</u>

- Protein: 16g
- Carbs: 5g
- Fats: 20g
- Calories: 255

Feisty Salad Of A Chicken

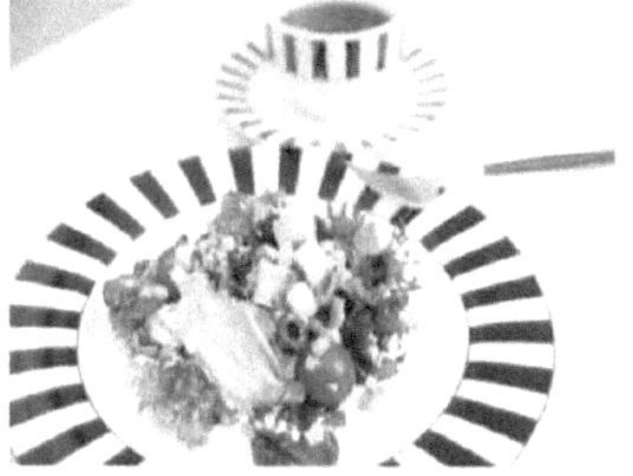

Serving: 2

Prep Time: 5 minutes

Cook Time: 30 minutes

Ingredients

- 1 whole piece of chicken
- 1 cup of water
- 1 cup of sour cream
- 1 teaspoon of garlic powder
- 1 teaspoon of black pepper
- 3 cup of baby spinach
- 3 diced up tomatoes
- 1 sliced up avocado

Process

1. The first step is to open up you're the lid of your instant pot and pour in water in your inner pot
2. Toss in your chicken
3. Set the instant pot on poultry mode and let it cook at high pressure for about 30 minutes
4. While that is being cooked, prepare your salad by taking a bowl and toss in the tomatoes, spinach, avocado and finely mix it
5. Toss in your sour cream alongside garlic powder, sprinkled with black pepper
6. By this time, the chicken should be ready. Open up your instant pot and bring it out, only to cut it finely

7. Once cut up, pour in your dressing and serve it warm over your prepared salad.

Nutrition

- Calories: 417
- Fat: 31g
- Carbohydrates: 2.55g
- Protein: 29g

Coolest Sausage Casserole

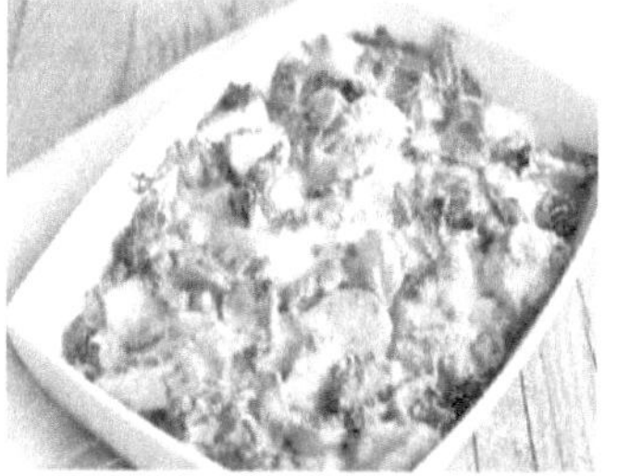

Serving: 6

Prep Time: 10 minutes

Cook Time: 30 minutes

Ingredients

- 1 pound of pork sausage
- 2 cups of diced up zucchini
- 2 cups of shredded green cabbage
- ½ a cup of diced up onion
- 3 pieces of large eggs
- ½ a cup of mayonnaise
- 2 teaspoon of yellow mustard
- 1 teaspoon of dried ground sage
- 1 and a ½ cup of shredded and divided cheddar cheese
- Cayenne pepper as required

How To

1. The first step here is to pre-heat your oven to a temperature of 375 degrees Fahrenheit
2. Take the casserole dish and grease it properly
3. Toss in the sausages over a large sized skillet and cook them over medium heat until a brown texture has appeared
4. Toss in the zucchini, onion, cabbages and let them cook until a tender feel has appeared
5. Turn off the heat and gently spoon into the casserole dish and finely keep it aside
6. Take a mixing bowl and toss in the whisk eggs, mayonnaise, sage and

pepper until a smooth texture has appeared

7. Toss in just 1 cup of the grated cheese into the egg mixture and finely stir
8. To the casserole with the remaining amount of cheese finely
9. Insert the prepared casserole into the pre-heated oven and let it bake for 30 minutes
10. After 30 minutes, take out the casserole after the cheese has melted down
11. Gently remove the roll from the oven and serve it hot

<u>Nutrition Values (Per Serving)</u>

- Protein: 19.11g
- Carbs: 6.12g
- Fats: 41g
- Calories: 487

The Ultimate Corned Beef With Cabbage

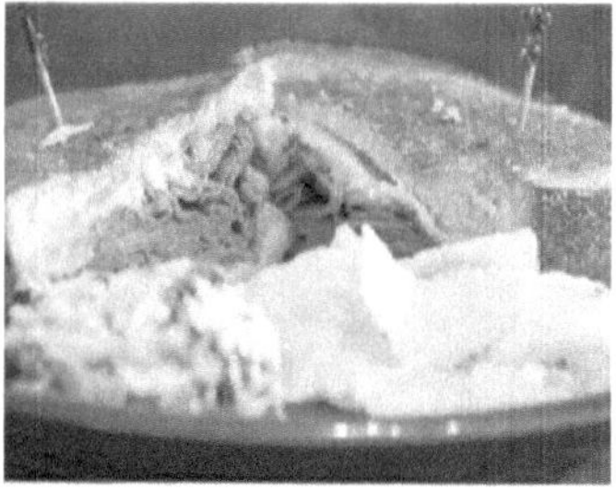

Serving: 4

Prep Time: 5 minutes

Cook Time: 120 minutes

<u>Ingredients</u>

- 1 piece of corned beef brisket
- 4 cups of water
- 1 small sized peeled and quartered onion
- 3 cloves of peeled and smashed garlic clove
- 2 pieces of bay leaves
- 3 whole sized black peppercorns
- ½ a teaspoon of allspice berries
- 1 teaspoon of dried thyme
- 5 medium sized carrots
- 1 head of a cabbage cut into wedges

<u>Process</u>

1. First step is to toss in the corned beef, onion, water, garlic cloves, allspice, peppercorn and thymes into your instant pot and close down the lid and set the timer to 90 minutes
2. Once the cooking is complete, turn off your device and allow the pressure to be excreted naturally.
3. Gently take out the meat and place them on a plate, only to cover them up with a tin foil and let it sit for just 15 minutes
4. Toss in the carrots and cabbage to the pot and lock up the lid, letting it cook for 10 minutes

5. Once the cooking is done, release the pressure quickly and take out the prepared vegetables and serve them alongside the corned beef.

Nutrition

- Calories: 478
- Fat: 25
- Carbohydrates: 3.8g
- Protein: 34.2g

Fluffy Ketogenic Donuts

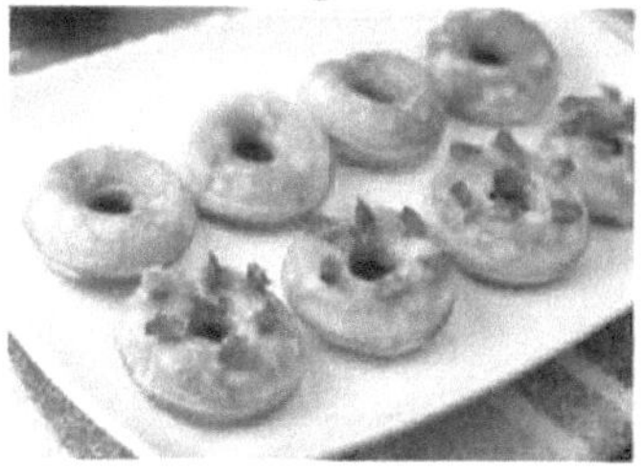

Serving: 22

Prep Time: 10 minutes

Cook Time: 35 minutes

Ingredients

- 1 cup of Golden Flaxseed Meal
- ¼ cup of cocoa powder
- 1 tablespoon of Cinnamon
- ½ tablespoon of Baking Powder
- ½ a teaspoon of Salt
- 1 piece of large egg
- 2 tablespoon of Coconut Oil
- ¼ cup of Sugar-free Caramel Syrup
- ½ a cup of Pumpkin Puree
- 1 teaspoon of Vanilla Extract
- 1 teaspoon of Apple Cider Vinegar
- ¼ cup of Silvered Almond

How To

1. The first step is to prepare your oven and pre-heat it to a temperature of 350 degrees Fahrenheit
2. Take a mixing bowl and toss in all of the ingredients in the bowl and combine everything
3. Take a muff tin and line it up with 6 paper liners
4. Scoop up the fill up the about ¼ of each of muffin liner
5. Sprinkle a bit of almond on top of the batter
6. Put it in your oven and let it bake for about 15 minutes
7. Once done, serve warm

Nutrition

- Calories: 183
- Fat: 13g
- Carbohydrates: 9g
- Protein: 7g

Creative Miniature Morning Pancakes

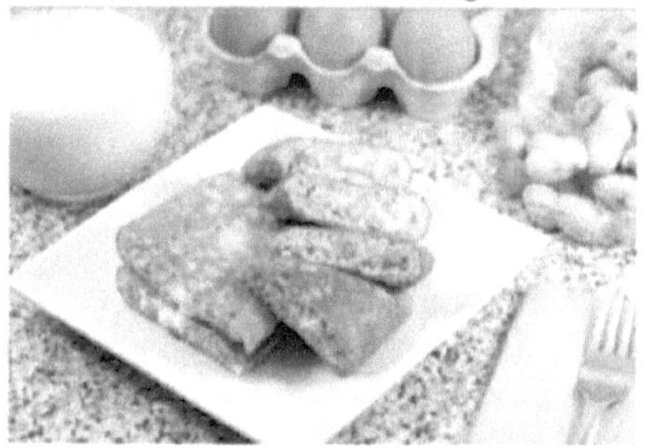

Serving: 2

Prep Time: 5 minutes

Cook Time: 10 minutes

Ingredients

For the Peanut Filling

- 1.8 ounce of Fresh Shelled Peanuts
- ½ a teaspoon of Stevia
- Salt as needed

For the Condensed Milk

- ¼ cup of Heavy cream
- 2 drops of Liquid Sucralose

For the Apam Balik

- ½ a cup of Almond Flour
- ½ a teaspoon of Bicarbonate Soda
- ½ a teaspoon of Baking Powder
- 1/8 teaspoon of Salt
- ¼ cup of Almond Milk
- 1 large sized Egg
- 5 drops of Liquid Sucralose
- ½ a teaspoon of Vanilla Extract
- ¼ teaspoon of coconut oil
- 1 tablespoon of Unsalted Butter

How To

1. The first step is to roast up your peanuts and brown them
2. Grind the peanuts alongside the salt and stevia to season it
3. Heat up your heavy cream and sucralose until a nice thick milk has formed
4. Take a mixing bowl and toss in the almond flour, baking powder, salt and baking soda. Mix them.
5. Then in that mixture, pour in the egg sucralose, vanilla extract, almond milk and egg. Mix again
6. Take a pan and melt your coconut oil, and pour in about half of the pancake mix
7. Cover it for about 1 minute and sprinkle in the ground peanuts and spread half of the condensed milk and butter
8. Cover the pan until cooked
9. Repeat until the whole batter is used.

Nutrition(Per Serving)

- Calories: 593
- Fat: 50g
- Carbohydrates: 11g
- Protein: 16g

Chapter 2: Lunch Recipes

Braised Beef Bone Short Ribs (Yummy!)

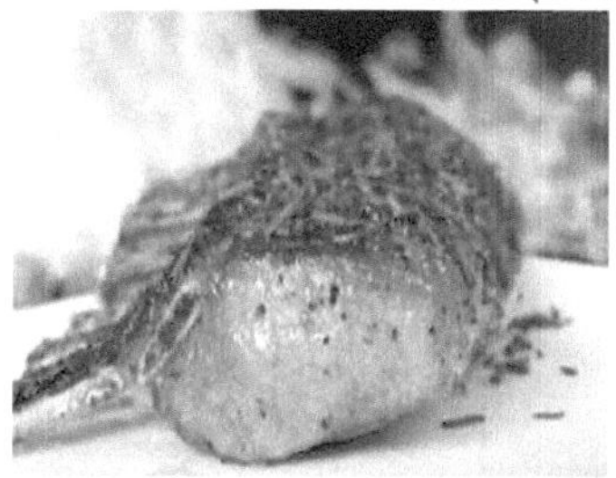

Serving: 5

Prep Time: 10 minutes

Cook Time: 35 minutes

Ingredients

- 4 pound of beef short ribs
- Generous amount of Kosher Salt
- 1 tablespoon of beef fat
- 1 quartered onion with its skin on
- 3 cloves of garlic
- Water

Process

1. Before beginning the cooking, you should first properly season the ribs with your preferred amount of salt
2. Take a skillet and heat up the beef oil over medium high. Toss in the ribs and gently cook them until browned
3. Once browned, toss in the garlic, onion and about 2 inches of water.
4. Once mixed, transfer the mixture to the instant pot and let it cook for about 35 minutes
5. Once the ribs complete, serve the dish with the dish on the bone
6. Alternatively, you can also pull the meat from the bones and braise the liquid and skim the fat. Store them in a jar and serve the ribs with the broth making sure to season them well.

Nutrition

- Calories: 550
- Fat: 39g
- Carbohydrates: 4g
- Protein: 14g

Crazy Homemade Bolognese

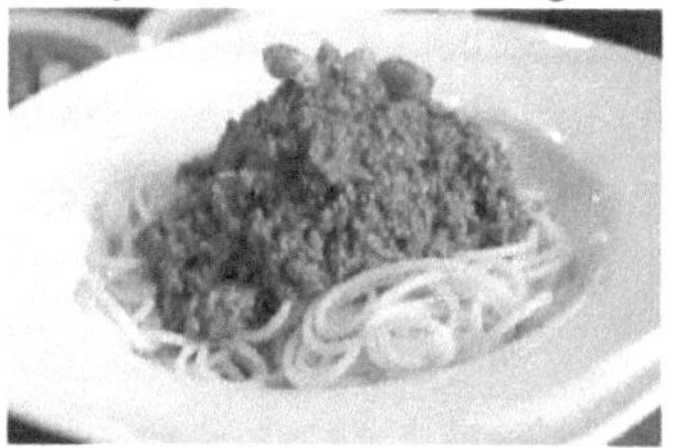

Serving: 4

Prep Time: 30 minutes

Cook Time: 10 minutes

Ingredients

- 4 tablespoon of olive oil
- 1 and a ½ cup of finely chopped onion
- ¾ cup of finely chopped carrots
- ¾ cup of finely chopped celery
- 2 tablespoon of minced garlic
- ½ a pound of spicy Italian pork sausage
- ½ a pound of ground chunk
- 1 and a ½ teaspoon of kosher salt
- ¾ teaspoon of black pepper
- 2 teaspoon of ground fennel
- 1 teaspoon of Italian seasoning
- ½ a cup of red wine
- 1 can of crushed tomatoes
- 1 tablespoon of sugar
- 1 pound of cooked pasta
- Parmesan cheese

Process

1. This recipe is very straightforward and will only require you to set your pot to Saute Mode and pour in the oil
2. Toss in the carrots, onions, celery, garlic and Saute them nicely
3. Toss in the ground meat then followed by the seasoning and let it

cook until the meat is perfectly browned up

4. Deglaze the pot with wine and cook for about 15 minutes
5. Stir while pouring tossing the tomatoes and sugar
6. Lock up the lid and let it cook at high pressure for 15 minutes
7. Once done, serve with spaghetti with sprinkles of parmesan cheese

Nutrition

- Calories: 237
- Fat: 14g
- Carbohydrates: 14g
- Protein: 16g

Super Cool Nasi Lemak

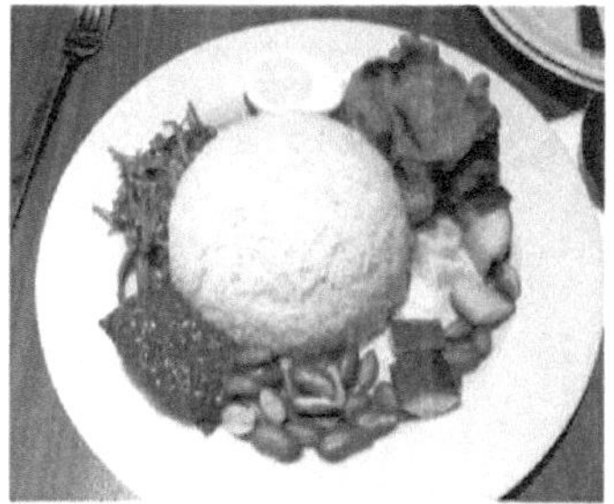

Serving: 1

Prep Time: 5 minutes

Cook Time: 5 minutes

Ingredients

- 3 ounce cream cheese
- 3 pieces of large eggs
- 4 tablespoon of Almond Flour
- 1 tablespoon of Coconut Flour
- 1 teaspoon of Baking powder
- 1 teaspoon of Vanilla Extract
- 4 tablespoon of Erythritol
- 10 drops of Liquid Stevia

How To

1. The first step is to toss in all of the ingredients in a bowl and mix them properly using an immersion blender
2. Open up your donut maker and spray it with coconut oil. Pour down the batter on the donut maker
3. Let it cook for about 3 minutes and flip them, let it cook for a more 2 minutes
4. Remove the donuts from the maker and let them cool. Repeat if any batter is left

Nutrition Values(Per Serving)

- Protein: 1.4g

- Carbs: 0.7g
- Fats: 2.7g
- Calories: 32

Wow! Crusted Salmon

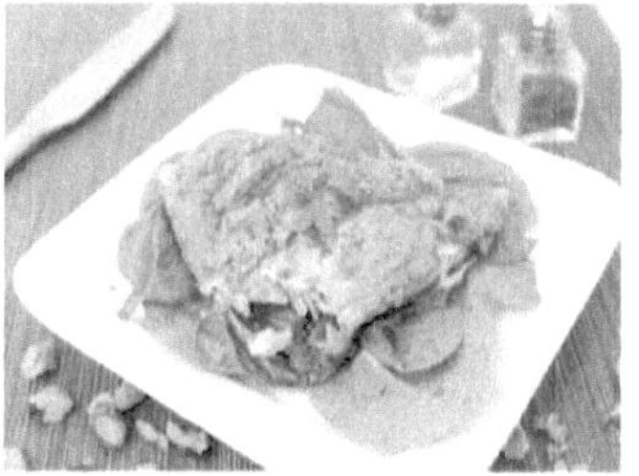

Serving: 2

Prep Time: 5 minutes

Cook Time: 8 minutes

Ingredients

- ½ a cup of walnuts
- 2 tablespoon of sugar-free maple syrup
- ½ a tablespoon of Dijon Mustard
- ¼ teaspoon of Dill
- 2 pieces of 3 ounce Salmon Fillets
- 1 tablespoon of Olive Oil
- Salt as needed
- Pepper as needed

How To

1. The first step is to preheat your oven to a temperature of 350 degrees Fahrenheit
2. Toss in the walnuts and pour the mustard and syrup into a food processor
3. Finely pulse it until a pasty consistency is achieved
4. Take a frying pan and heat it up with a good amount of oil until extremely hot
5. Take your salmon and toss them into the pan and sear them for 3 minutes
6. While It is being seared, toss in the walnut mixture on the top side of the salmon

7. Transfer it to your oven and bake for 8 minutes
8. Serve hot

Nutrition Values(Per Serving)

- Protein: 20g
- Carbs: 4g
- Fats: 43g
- Calories: 373

Hot And Warm Jalapeno Popper Mug Cake

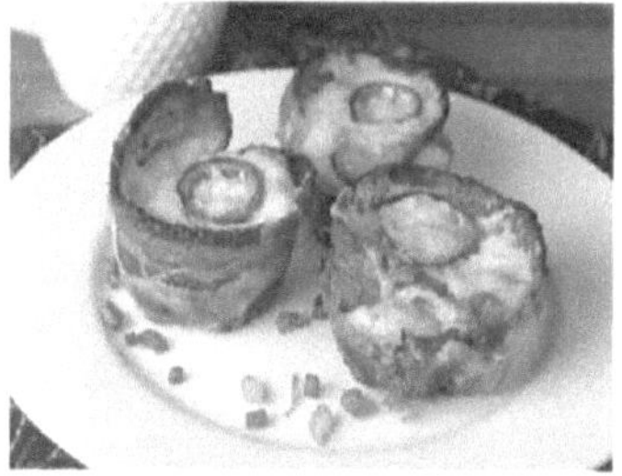

Serving: 1

Prep Time: 5 minutes

Cook Time: 5 minutes

Ingredients

- 2 tablespoon of Almont Flour
- 1 tablespoon of Golden Flaxseed Meal
- 1 tablespoon of Butter
- 1 tablespoon of Cream Cheese
- 1 large side Egg
- 1 sliced and cooked bacon
- ½ of a Jalapeno Pepper
- ½ teaspoon of Baking Powder
- ¼ teaspoon of Salt

How To

1. Take a frying pan and place it over medium heat.
2. Take the sliced bacon and cook it until it has a crispy texture
3. Take a container and mix all of the ingredients together
4. Clean the sides
5. Microwave the whole dish for 75 seconds putting it on power 10
6. Gently slam out the cup against a plate to take out the mug cake out
7. Garnish it with some jalapeno and serve it

Nutrition Values(Per Serving)

- Protein: 16.5g

- Carbs: 8.4g
- Fats: 38g
- Calories: 429

Fantastic Ham Stromboli

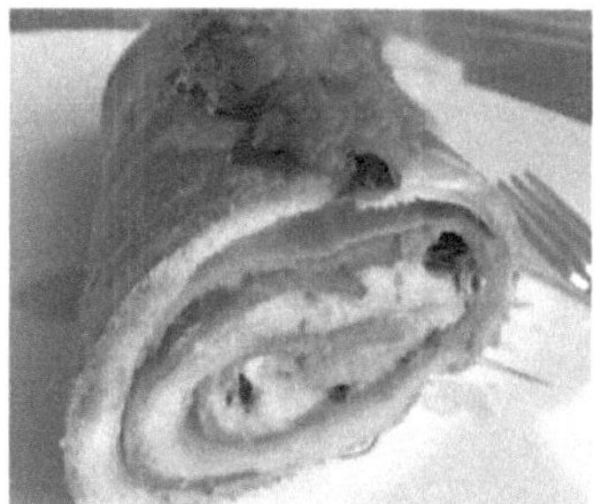

Serving: 4

Prep Time: 6 minutes

Cook Time: 20 minutes

Ingredients

- 1 and a quarter cup of shredded mozzarella cheese
- 4 tablespoon of almond flour
- 3 tablespoon of coconut flour
- 1 large sized egg
- 1 teaspoon of Italian seasoning
- 14 ounce of Ham
- 3 and a half ounce of Cheddar Cheese
- Salt as required
- Pepper as required

How To

1. Pre-heat your oven to a temperature of 400 degrees Fahrenheit and melt up your mozzarella cheese in a microwave oven

2. Take mixing a bowl and toss in the coconut flour, almond flour and seasoning and mix them properly

3. Then pour in the melted mozzarella cheese and keep mixing

4. After a minute, the cheese will be cooled down and here toss in your egg and mix everything again

5. Once combined, take a fine parchment paper and on a flat surface transfer the mixture

6. Take a rolling pin to flatten it out evenly

7. Take a pizza cutter and cut diagonal lines in the dough from the edges going all the way to the center

8. Make sure that you leave about 4 inches wide rows of the dough untouched in between

9. Between the diagonal layers, fill it up with ham and cheddar

10. Once done, leave a section of the dough and roll it on top of another. Completely covering the filling

11. Finally, bake it for about 15-20 minutes and serve when a nice golden brown texture has appeared

<u>Nutrition Values(Per Serving)</u>

- Protein: 25.6g
- Carbs: 8.5g
- Fats: 21.8g
- Calories: 305.5

A Delicious Pepper and Sausage Soup

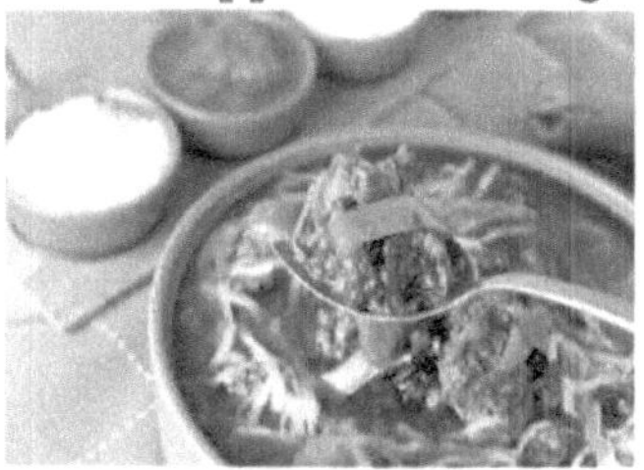

Serving: 2

Prep Time: 10 minutes

Cook Time: 45 minutes

Ingredients

- 32 ounce of Pork Sausages
- 1 tablespoon of Olive Oil
- 10 ounce of Raw Spinach
- 1 medium sized Green Bell Pepper
- 1 can of jalapenos with tomatoes
- 4 cup of beef stock
- 1 tablespoon of chili powder
- 1 tablespoon of cumin
- 1 teaspoon of Garlic Powder
- 1 teaspoon of Italian Seasoning
- ¾ teaspoon of Salt

How To

1. The first step is to take a large pot and heat your olive oil over medium heat
2. Toss in the sausages and cook them until seared fine. Stir everything.
3. Slice up the green pepper into fine pieces and toss them to the pot as well
4. Season it with salt and pepper
5. Toss in the tomatoes and jalapenos and mix once more
6. Toss in the spinach on top of everything and close up the lid. Once

the spinach is wilted, add in the rest of the spices and broth

7. Close the lid and keep it covered for about 30 minutes over medium-low heat.
8. Once done, remove the lid and simmer it for 15 minutes and you are done.

<u>Nutrition Values(Per Serving)</u>

- Protein: 27g
- Carbs: 3.8g
- Fats: 2.3g
- Calories: 525

The Genius Reversed Bacon Burger

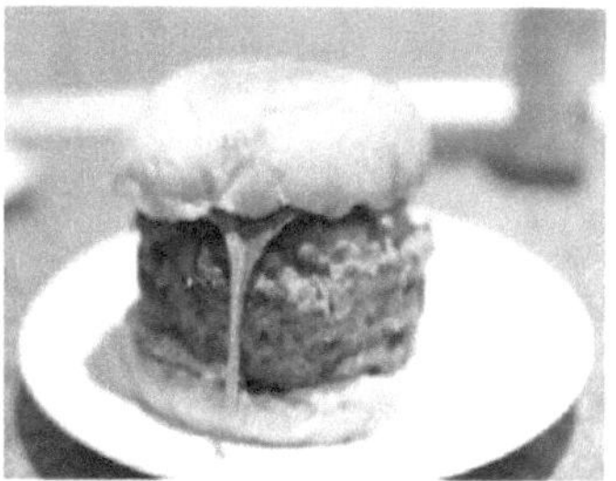

Serving: 2

Prep Time: 10 minutes

Cook Time: 15 minutes

Ingredients

- 800g of Ground Beef
- 8 slices of Chopped up Bacon
- ¼ cup of cheddar cheese
- 2 tablespoon of chopped up Chives
- 2 teaspoon of Minced Garlic
- 2 teaspoon of Black Pepper
- 1 tablespoon of Soy Sauce
- 1 and a ¼ teaspoon of Salt
- 1 teaspoon of Onion Powder
- 1 teaspoon of Worcestershire Sauce

How To

1. Take a cast iron skillet and cook up all of your chopped bacon until a fine crispy texture has appeared
2. Once done, remove and place them on a kitchen towel
3. Drain the grease for later use
4. Take a large mixing bowl and toss in the ground beef, 2/3 of chopped up Bacon and the spices
5. Mix the meat finely alongside the spices and form 9 patties
6. Put about 2 tablespoons of Bacon Fat into the cast iron and place the patties once the fat is considerably hot
7. Let them cook for about 4-5 minutes with batches of 3-4

8. Remove them, cool for 5 minutes and top it off with some extra bacon, onion or cheese

<u>Nutrition Values(Per Serving)</u>

- Protein: 174g
- Carbs: 7g
- Fats: 207g
- Calories: 2597

Chapter 3: Dinner Recipes

Delicious Shrimp Curry Alongside Peanuts

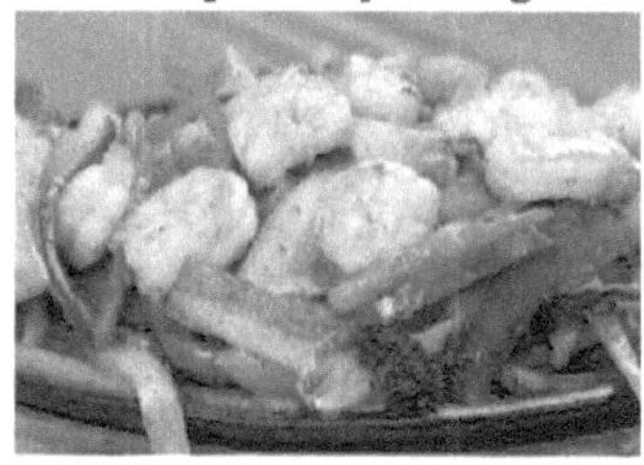

Serving: 2

Prep Time: 5 minutes

Cook Time: 10 minutes

<u>Ingredients</u>

- 2 tablespoon of Green Curry Paste
- 1 cup of vegetable stock
- 1 cup of coconut milk
- 6 ounce of Pre-Cooked Shrimp
- 5 ounce of Broccoli florets
- 3 tablespoon of chopped Cilantro
- 2 tablespoon of Coconut Oil
- 1 tablespoon of Peanut Butter
- 1 tablespoon of Soy Sauce
- ½ of a lime juice
- 1 medium sized spring onion chopped up
- 1 teaspoon of crushed roasted garlic
- 1 teaspoon of minced garlic
- 1 teaspoon of fish sauce
- ½ teaspoon of Turmeric
- ¼ teaspoon of Xanthan Gum
- ½ of a cup of source cream

<u>How To</u>

1. Start up by taking a pan over medium heat and add up 2 tablespoons of coconut oil

2. Once the oil is melted toss in the minced ginger and chopped up spring onion. Let them cook for about a minute before pouring the turmeric and curry paste

3. Add about 1 tablespoon of soy sauce, peanut butter and fish sauce and mix them well

4. Then add in a cup of vegetable stock and just a cup of coconut milk.

5. Stir them well before adding the green curry paste.

6. Simmer them for a while

7. Add in about ¼ teaspoon of Xanthan Gum to the curry and mix it properly

8. After a while you will notice that the curry will begin to thicken, that will be the moment when you are going to be needing to throw in the florets and stir them finely

9. Add in the fresh chopped cilantro

10. Once the consistency is fine, you are going to need to toss the weighed pre-cooked shrimp and add the lime juice

11. Let the mixture for a few minutes and season it with pepper and salt as required

12. Finally, serve it hot alongside just a ¼ a cup of sour cream with each serving

<u>Nutrition Values(Per Serving)</u>

- Protein: 27g
- Carbs: 8.9g
- Fats: 31g
- Calories: 454

The Original Keto Sushi

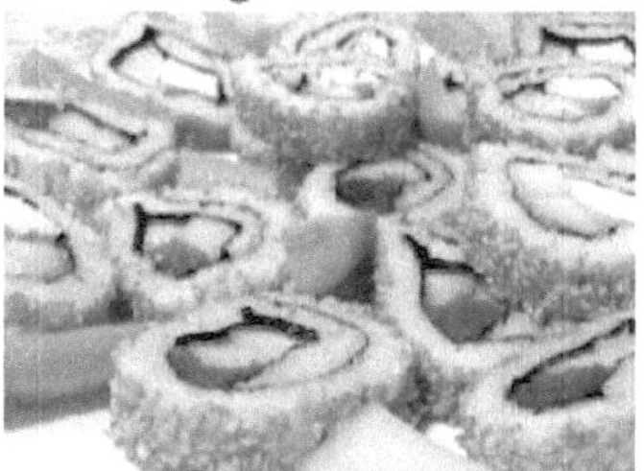

Serving: 3

Prep Time: 10 minutes

Cook Time: 10 minutes

Ingredients

- 16 ounce of cauliflower
- 6 ounce of softened cream cheese
- 1-2 tablespoon of Rice Vinegar
- 1 tablespoon of Soy Sauce
- 5 sheets of Nori
- 1 piece of 6-inch cucumber
- ½ a piece of medium Avocado
- 5 ounce of smoked salmon

How To

1. Take a food processor and rice up the cauliflower into rice-sized pieces
2. Take a cucumber and slice it up on each end
3. Gently place the cucumber upright and slice off the sides
4. Finely discard the middle part and slice about 2 pieces into small strips
5. Keep it in a fridge
6. Take a skillet and heat it up, toss in the rice and cook it up
7. Season it with soy sauce
8. Once the cooking is complete, toss the cauliflower into a bowl and mix the cream cheese alongside the rice vinegar
9. Mix well and set it in the fridge

10. Once the mixture is cooled, slice about ½ of your avocado and scoop out small strips out of the shell

11. Take your nori sheet down a bamboo roller and cover it with saran wrap

12. Spread out some cauliflower rice over the nori sheets, toss in the fillings and roll up tightly before serving

<u>Nutrition Values (Per Serving)</u>

- Protein: 18g
- Carbs: 5.7g
- Fats: 25g
- Calories: 353

Great Pumpkin Carbonara

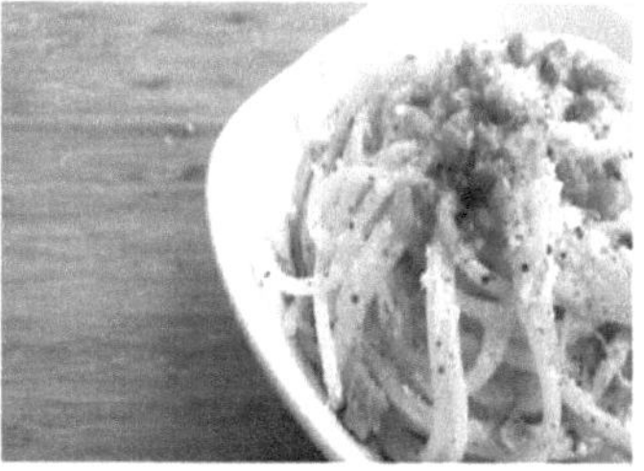

Serving: 3

Prep Time: 10 minutes

Cook Time: 10 minutes

Ingredients

- 1 package of Shirataki Noodles
- 5 ounce of Pancetta
- 2 large sized Egg Yolks
- ¼ cup of heavy cream
- 1/3 cup of Parmesan Cheese
- 2 tablespoon of Butter
- 3 tablespoon of Pumpkin Puree
- ½ teaspoon of Dried Sage
- Salt as needed
- Pepper as needed

How To

1. The first step here is to rise off your noodles in hot water for about 2-3 minutes and dry them completely

2. Chop up your pancetta place them in a hot pan.

3. Sear them on the outside and let them get a crispy texture

4. Once done, remove them from the pan and store the fat

5. Take another hot pan and toss in the butter and let it brown

6. Once browned enough, pour in the pumpkin puree and sage

7. Pour in the heavy cream and fat to the mixture and finely mix everything

8. Turn the heat to high and toss in the noodles. Dry fry them for about 5

minutes, you should get a considerable amount of steam.

9. Toss in the parmesan cheese to the pumpkin sauce and mix everything finely

10. Lower down the heat and keep stirring it until a fine thick sauce is produced

11. Toss in the noodles and pancetta into the prepared sauce and toss them well

12. Finally, to top everything off, add in 2 egg yolks and mix them into the sauce

<u>Nutrition Values(Per Serving)</u>

- Protein: 14g
- Carbs: 2g
- Fats: 34g
- Calories: 384
- Fiber: 2g

A Chicken Sandwich Filled With Bacon and Avocado

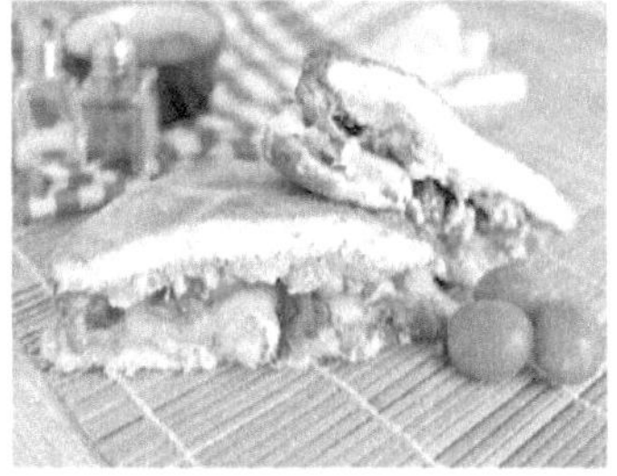

Serving: 2

Prep Time: 10 minutes

Cook Time: 25 minutes

Ingredients

Required for the Cloud Bread

- 3 large pieces of eggs
- 3 ounce of cream cheese
- 1/8 teaspoon of tartar cream
- ¼ teaspoon of salt
- ½ teaspoon of garlic powder

Required for the filling

- 1 tablespoon of mayonnaise
- 1 teaspoon of Sriracha
- 2 Bacon slices
- 3 ounce of Chicken
- 2 pepper jack cheese slices
- 2 grape tomatoes
- ¼ of a medium sized avocado

How To

1. First, pre-heat your oven to a temperature of 300 degrees Fahrenheit
2. Take three different bowls and crack in the eggs individually
3. Toss in the tartar cream to one bowl alongside some salt and keep whipping until a nice foamy texture appears

4. In another bowl, keep beating the yolk and add in the cream cheese until a fine pale yellow color has appeared
5. Gently pour the egg whites into yolk mixture
6. Take a parchment paper lined baking sheet and scoop about ¼ cup of the prepared batter
7. Finely form them into square shapes and sprinkle just a bit of garlic
8. Bake for 25 minutes
9. On the side, cook the bacon and chicken by seasoning them with some pepper and finally ready the sandwich using the mixture, mayo, halved tomato, mashed avocado, sriracha and cheese.

<u>Nutrition Values(Per Serving)</u>

- Protein: 22g
- Carbs: 4g
- Fats: 28g
- Calories: 361

Juicy And Cheesy Molten Bites

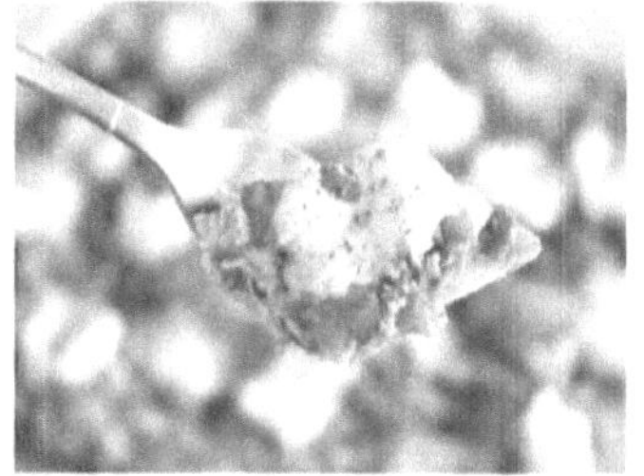

Serving: 2

Prep Time: 10 minutes

Cook Time: 10 minutes

Ingredients

- 10 ounce of Drained up Canned Tuna
- ¼ cup of mayonnaise
- 1 cubed and medium sized Avocado
- ¼ cup of Parmesan Cheese
- 1/3 cup of Almond Flour
- ½ teaspoon of Garlic Powder
- ¼ teaspoon of Onion Powder
- Salt as needed
- Pepper as needed
- ½ a cup of Coconut Oil

How To

1. The first step here is to take a mixing bowl and toss in all of the listed ingredients with the exclusion of the coconut oil and avocado
2. Take the cubed avocado and fold them into the tuna
3. Finely fold tuna into balls and cover them up with Almond Flour
4. Take a pan and pour the coconut oil and heat it up over medium heat
5. Toss in the tuna balls and fry them until a nice brown texture has appeared
6. Serve hot

Nutrition Values(Per Serving)

- Protein: 6.2g
- Carbs: 2.0g
- Fats: 11.8g
- Calories: 134

A Romantic Low Carb Chicken Satay

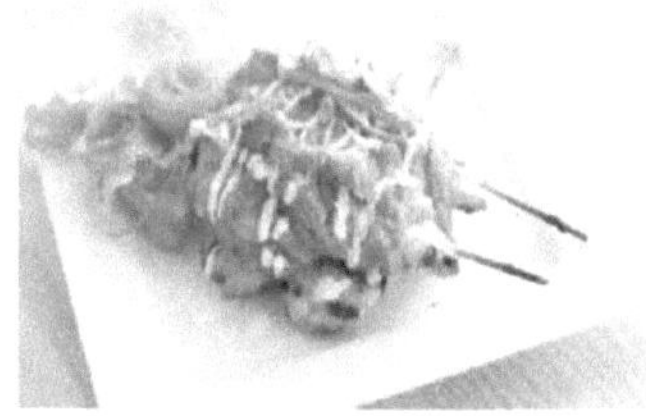

Serving: 1

Prep Time: 5 minutes

Cook Time: 5 minutes

Ingredients

- 1 pound of Ground Chicken
- 4 tablespoon of Soy Sauce
- 3 tablespoon of Peanut Butter
- 2 springs of Onion
- 1/3 pieces of Yellow Pepper
- 1 tablespoon of Erythritol
- 1 tablespoon of Rice Vinegar
- 2 teaspoon of Sesame Oil
- 2 teaspoon of Chili Paste
- 1 teaspoon of Minced Garlic
- 1/3 teaspoon of Cayenne Pepper
- ¼ teaspoon of Paprika
- Juice of ½ a lime

How To

1. Heat up about 2 teaspoons of your sesame oil on medium high-heat pan
2. Brown up your chicken and toss in all of the ingredients. Finely mix them and keep cooking
3. Once cooked, toss in about 2 chopped up spring onions and 1/3 of your sliced yellow pepper
4. Serve hot

<u>**Nutrition Values(Per Serving)**</u>

- Protein: 105g
- Carbs: 18g
- Fats: 69g
- Calories: 1180

Traditional Salmon Glazed With Sesame And Ginger

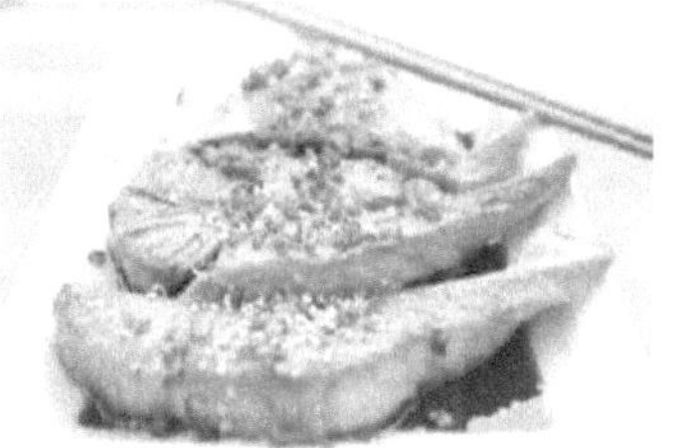

Serving: 2

Prep Time: 10 minutes

Cook Time: 10 minutes

Ingredients

- 10 ounce of Salmon Fillet
- 2 tablespoon of Soy Sauce
- 2 teaspoon of Sesame Oil
- 1 tablespoon of Rice Vinegar
- 1 teaspoon of Minced Ginger
- 2 teaspoon of Minced Garlic
- 1 tablespoon of Red boat Fish Sauce
- 1 tablespoon of Sugar-Free Ketchup
- 2 tablespoon of White Wine

How To

1. Toss in all of the ingredients to a small sized Tupperware. Just make sure not to toss the sesame oil, white wine, and ketchup

2. Marinade everything for about 10-15 minutes

3. Bring down the pan to a nice heat and toss in the sesame oil

4. One the smoke is seen, toss the fish with the skin side down

5. Let it cook until crispy

6. Flip it and cook the other side

7. Each side should take about 3-4 minutes

8. Pour in the marinade liquid to the fish and let it boil

9. Slowly remove the fish from the pan and pour in the ketchup alongside the white wine to the liquid in the pan

10. Simmer for 5 minutes and serve as a side

Nutrition Values(Per Serving)

- Protein: 33g
- Carbs: 2.5g
- Fats: 23.5g
- Calories: 370

Cilantro Paste With A Whole Lot Of Skirt Steak

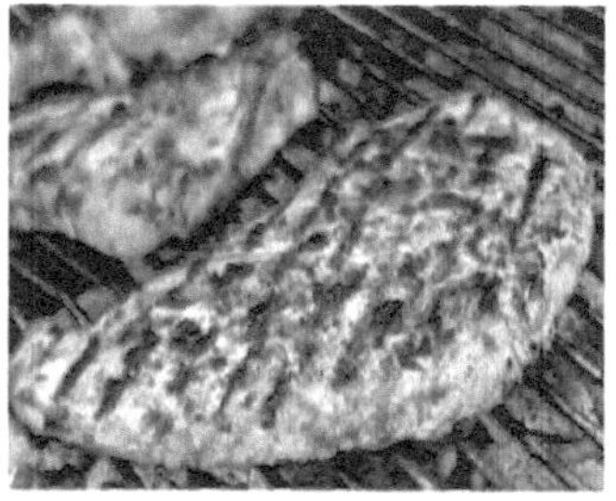

Serving: 3

Prep Time: 45 minutes

Cook Time: 10 minutes

Ingredients

For the Cilantro Lime Steak Marinade

- 1 pound of Skirt Steak
- ¼ cup of Soy Sauce
- ¼ cup of Olive Oil
- 1 medium sized lime completely juiced
- 1 teaspoon of Minced Garlic
- 1 small sized Handful Cilantro
- ¼ teaspoon of Red Pepper Flakes

For the Cilantro Paste

- 1 teaspoon of Minced Garlic
- ½ a teaspoon of Salt
- 1 cup of lightly fresh cilantro
- ¼ cup of olive oil
- ½ a medium sized juiced lemon
- 1 medium sized deseeded Jalapeno
- ½ a teaspoon of Cumin
- ½ a teaspoon of Coriander

How To

1. The first step here is to remove outer silver skin off your skirt steak

and toss in all of the Cilantro Lime Steak marinade ingredients inside a plastic bag alongside the Steak
2. Let them marinate for about 45 minutes in a fridge
3. For the sauce, you need to toss in all the paste ingredients into a food processor and pulse them until finely blended
4. Take an iron skillet and put it over medium-high heat
5. Once heated up, toss in the steak to the pan and finely cook on either sides. It should not take more than 2-3 minutes per side

Nutrition Values(Per Serving)

- Protein: 32.3g
- Carbs: 2.8g
- Fats: 32.5g
- Calories: 432

Chapter 4: Snack Recipes

Delicious Stuffed Peppers

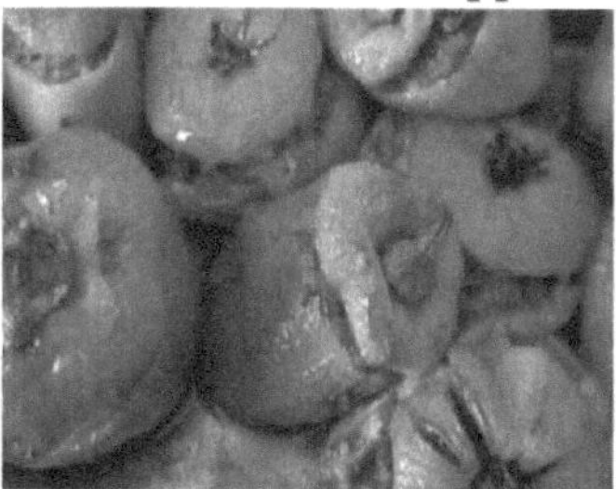

Serving: 4

Prep Time: 5 minutes

Cook Time: 16 minutes

Ingredients

- 4 red bell peppers with their tops cut off
- 1 cup of white bean soaked up overnight
- 1 cup of quinoa
- 1 cup of goat cheese
- 3 cups of vegetable broth
- 2 tablespoon of garlic powder

Process

1. Open up the lid of your pot and toss in the quinoa, beans, garlic powder and pour in the vegetable broth as well
2. Let it cook at high pressure for 8 minutes
3. Release the pressure naturally
4. Take your pepper and fill it up with bean and quinoa mixture
5. Wipe out your instant pot and place your filled in pepper in it
6. Change your instant pot mode to warm and keep it like that for 6 minutes.
7. Take it out and serve hot

Nutrition

- Calories: 313
- Fat: 24g
- Carbohydrates: 9g
- Protein: 15g

Cute Miniature Spiced Muffins

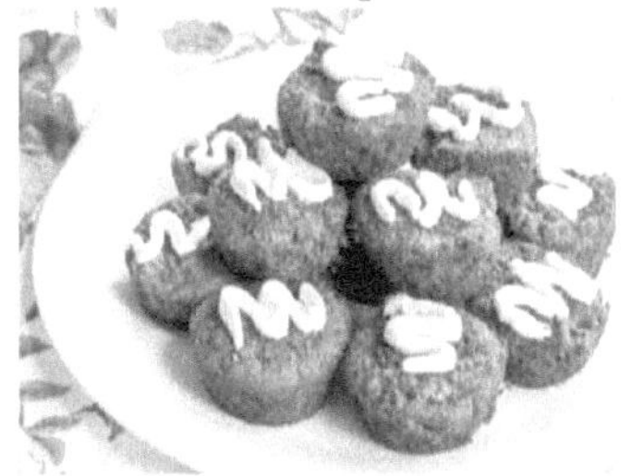

Serving: 18

Prep Time: 10 minutes

Cook Time: 15 minutes

Ingredients

- ¾ cup of canned of pumpkin
- ¼ of cup of organic seed butter
- 1 large of egg at room temperature
- 1/ cup of Erythritol
- ¼ cup of sifted organic coconut flour
- 2 tablespoon of organic flaxseed meal
- 1 teaspoon of ground cinnamon
- ½ a teaspoon of ground nutmeg
- ½ a teaspoon of baking soda
- ½ teaspoon of baking powder
- ¼ teaspoon of salt

How To

1. The first step here is to pre-heat your oven to a temperature of 350 degrees Fahrenheit
2. Take the muffin pan and lightly grease it up
3. Take a bowl and mix in the sunflower seed butter, pumpkin and egg. Keep stirring the whole mixture until a smooth consistency has been gained
4. Toss in all of the remaining ingredients and let it blend
5. Take a tablespoon-sized scoop and scoop up the batter and fill in the muffin sections

6. Place the tray inside the oven and let it cook for about 15 minutes
7. Once the timer runs out, gently remove the tray from the oven and top the muffins with cream cheese
8. Serve warm

Nutrition(Per Serving)

- Calories: 42
- Fat: 2.9g
- Carbohydrates: 1.23g
- Protein: 1.84g

Time Pass White Pizza Frittata

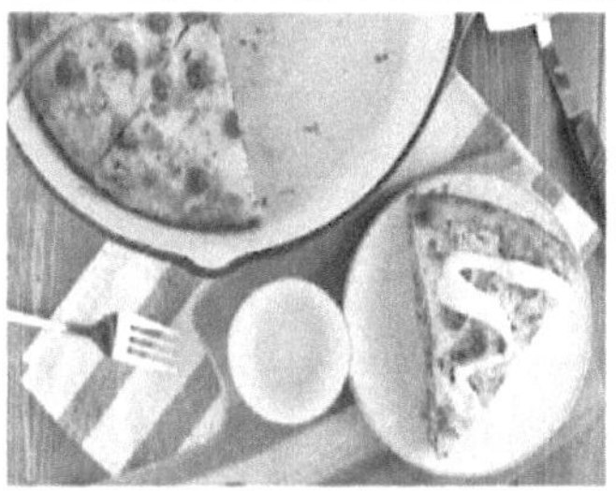

Serving: 18

Prep Time: 10 minutes

Cook Time: 30 minutes

Ingredients

- 12 large sized eggs
- 9 ounce of Frozen Spinach
- 1 ounce of pepperoni
- 5 ounce of Mozzarella Cheese
- 1 teaspoon of Minced up Garlic
- ½ a cup of parmesan Cheese
- 4 tablespoon of Olive Oil
- ¼ teaspoon of Nutmeg
- Salt as needed
- Pepper as needed

How To

1. Start off the recipe by microwaving your frozen spinach for about 3-4 minutes
2. Gently squeeze the spinaches later on to drain the water out
3. Pre-heat your oven to a temperature of 375 degrees.
4. Take a bowl and mix in the eggs, spices alongside the olive oil
5. Toss in the spinach, parmesan and ricotta
6. Take an iron skillet and pour in the prepared mixture
7. Sprinkle some mozzarella cheese and pepperoni
8. Put it in the oven and let it bake for 30 minutes before serving hot!

Nutrition(Per Serving)

- Calories: 298
- Fat: 23g
- Carbohydrates: 2.9g
- Protein: 19g

Mesmerizing Cheese Drizzled Zucchini Boats

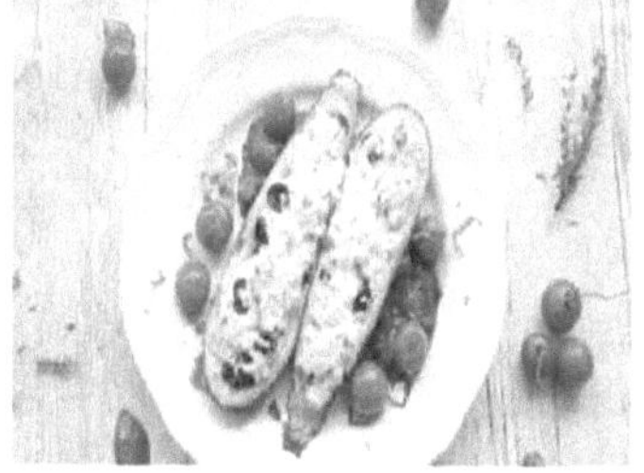

Serving: 4

Prep Time: 5 minutes

Cook Time: 16 minutes

Ingredients

- 3 tablespoon of olive oil
- 2 cup of zucchini
- 2 cups of spiralized carrots
- 3 chopped up garlic cloves
- 2 cups of vegetable broth
- 1 tablespoon of black pepper
- 1 tablespoon of garlic powder

Process

1. The first step is to toss in all of the ingredients in your instant pot
2. Cover up the lid and let it cook for about 4 minutes at high pressure
3. Once done, release the pressure naturally and serve it hot with some cheese sprinkled up

Nutrition

- Calories: 237
- Fat: 20g
- Carbohydrates: 7g
- Protein: 10g

The Simplest Sausage and Pepper Meal

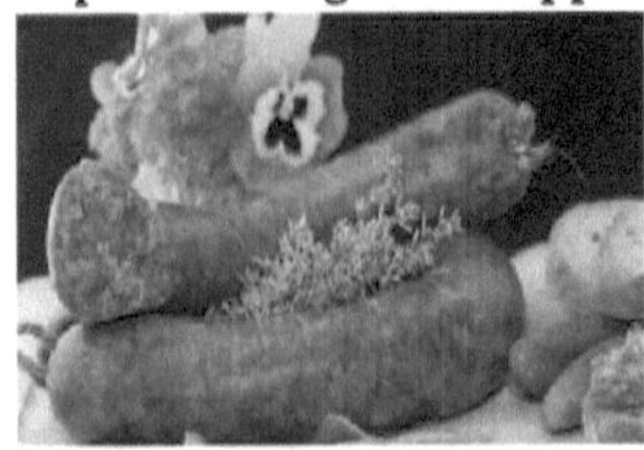

Serving: 3

Prep Time: 5 minutes

Cook Time: 10 minutes

Ingredients

- 2 pound of Italian Sausage
- 2 sliced up bell peppers
- 2 chopped up Zucchini
- 1 chopped up onion
- 28 ounce of Italian stewed tomatoes
- 16 ounce of pasta sauce
- ½ a pound of dry penne pasta
- 1 and a ½ tablespoon of Italian seasoning
- Grated Parmesan cheese

Process

1. Start off the recipe by removing the sausage meat from their personal casing and tossing them to your instant pot.
2. Saute them until nicely browned up
3. Drain out the fat from your cooker and toss in the garlic, peppers and onions and let it cook for another 3 minutes
4. Stir in the remaining ingredients and pour just enough water to cover the ingredients up
5. Lock up the lid and let it cook at high pressure for 8 minutes
6. Naturally, release the pressure and open the lid
7. Transfer the mixture to your serving plate and serve with grated parmesan as garnish

Nutrition

- Calories: 288
- Fat: 21g
- Carbohydrates: 9g
- Protein: 14g

Heart Warming Grandmother's Hot Chili Soup

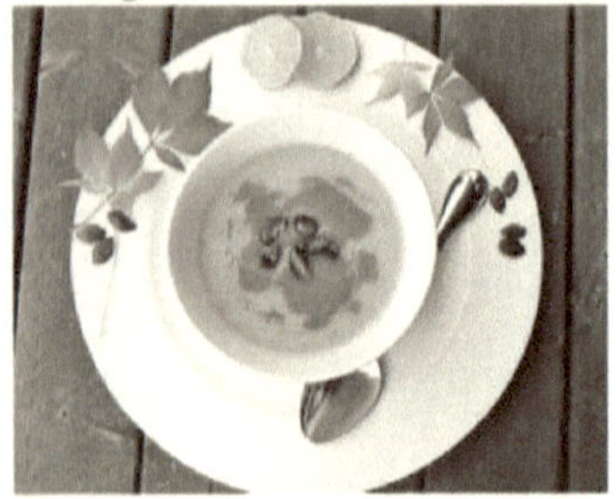

Serving: 5

Prep Time: 5 minutes

Cook Time: 10 minutes

Ingredients

- 1 teaspoon of Coriander Seeds
- 2 tablespoon of Olive Oil
- 2 sliced chili pepper
- 2 cups of chicken broth
- 2 cups of water
- 1 teaspoon of Turmeric
- ½ a teaspoon of Ground Cumin
- 4 tablespoon of Tomato Paste
- 16 ounce of chicken thigh
- 2 tablespoon of butter
- 1 medium sized avocado
- 2 ounce of Queso Fresco
- 4 tablespoon of chopped up Cilantro
- Juice of a half lime
- Salt as required
- Pepper as required

How To

1. Cut up your chicken thighs and finely place them in a cooking pan dipped with oil
2. Cook them until brown and place them on the side
3. A tin of about just 2 tablespoons of olive oil, toss in the coriander

seeds and heat them. Once the fragrance is out, toss in the chili,

4. Pour down the water and broth and let it finely simmer

5. Season the mixture with turmeric, pepper, salt and ground cumin

6. Once it has reached a simmering point, add in the tomato paste alongside the butter and stir it to combine and mix

7. Let it simmer for about 10 minutes

8. Pour in the juice

9. In your soup bowl, place about 4 ounces of chicken thighs and ladle it

10. Garnish finally with just ¼ of our avocado and serve it with an ounce of cilantro and queso fresco

<u>Nutrition Values(Per Serving)</u>

- Protein: 28g
- Carbs: 10.8g
- Fats: 27g
- Calories: 395

Excellent Chicken Roulades With Gruyere And Sage

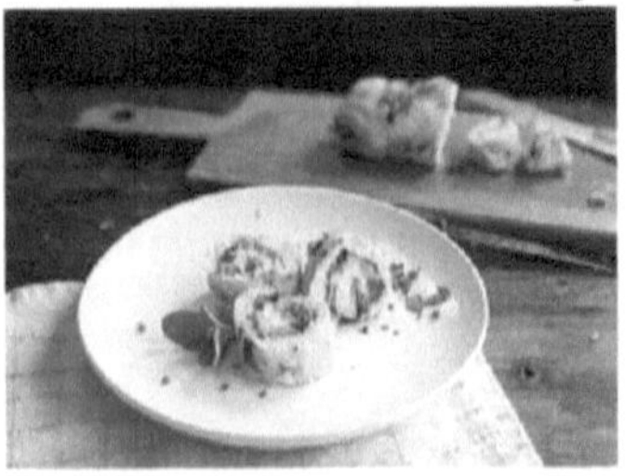

Serving: 5

Prep Time: 4 minutes

Cook Time: 40 minutes

Ingredients

- 2 pieces of chicken breast
- 1 tablespoon of butter
- 1 medium sized onion all diced up
- 1 tablespoon of white wine vinegar
- 3 ounce of finely grated Gruyere cheese
- 2 tablespoon and a 1 teaspoon of finely chopped fresh sage
- Salt as required
- Pepper as required

How To

1. The first step is to preheat your oven to 375 degrees Fahrenheit
2. Take an 11 x 13-inch baking pan and line it with parchment paper
3. Take the chicken breast and butterfly them. Take a nice knife and cut along the side of the breast in a sawing motion. Cut it similar to opening up a bagel
4. Make sure that you don't completely slice it off, open the breast and lay it flat
5. Sandwich each of the breasts between plastic wraps and beat it using a meat tenderizing mallet until they are flat at about ¼ inch thick
6. Season them with pepper and salt
7. Take a medium sized skillet and heat it over medium heat
8. Toss in the butter and let it foam. Toss in the onions and cook them

over until they are caramelized

9. Pour in the white wine vinegar and stir in until a syrupy consistency has formed.

10. Remove the heat and toss in the 2 tablespoons of sage and keep stirring it to combine

11. Season with just an amount of pepper and salt

12. Lay out about three pieces of twin and on top of them, place the flattened breast

13. Make sure that the filling is away from the edges, gently spread ½ of the onion mixture over each of the chicken breasts

14. Sprinkle about 2 ounces of grated cheese over the breast

15. Gently roll up the breasts and secure them using a twine

16. Take a baking pan and place them in it and sprinkle in the leftover sage and cheese over the roulades

17. Bake it for about 35 minutes

18. Remove and let it cool for 5 minutes and serve

<u>Nutrition Values(Per Serving)</u>

- Protein: 42g
- Carbs: 2g
- Fats: 14g
- Calories: 315

Faster Than Lightning Swift Kimchi

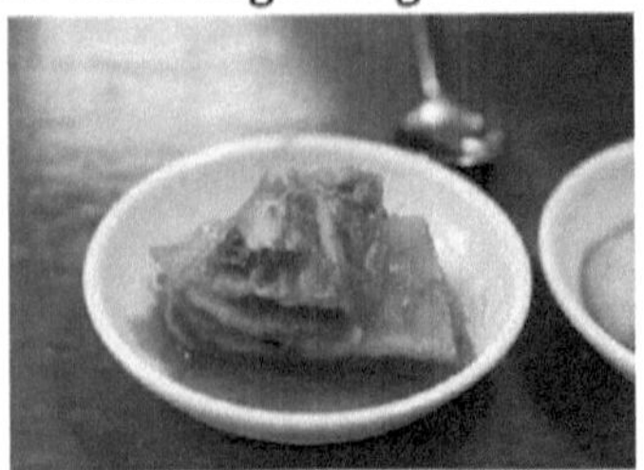

Serving: 4

Prep Time: 5 minutes

Cook Time: 10 minutes

Ingredients

For the Quick Kimchi

- 3 cups of Purple Cabbage
- 3 tablespoon of Rice Vinegar
- 1 tablespoon of Minced up Garlic
- 2 teaspoon of minced Ginger
- 1 and a ½ tablespoon of Red Pepper Flakes
- 1/3 of a medium Daikon Radish
- 1 large sized Scallion
- 1 medium sized red Chili
- 1 tablespoon of Red Curry Paste
- 1 and a ½ tablespoon of Soy Sauce

For the Stir Fry

- 1 pound of Pork Tenderloin
- 3 tablespoon of Coconut Oil
- 3 and a ½ ounce of Shitake Mushroom
- 1 large sized Scallion
- 2 tablespoon of White Wine
- 1 tablespoon of NOW Erythritol
- 2 tablespoon of Sesame Oil
- Salt as needed
- Pepper as needed

<u>**How To**</u>

1. Take your cabbage and slice it up into fine strips
2. Slice up your radish into matchstick sizes
3. Mix up all of the quick Kimchi ingredients in a bowl and combine well
4. Take your pork loin and slice it up to 1/4 inch thick medallions
5. Pour about 1 tablespoon of coconut oil to a pan and toss in half of the pork and cook it until brown spots appear on either sides
6. Repeat for the other half
7. Pour in the wine, 1 tablespoon of coconut oil alongside the sesame oil
8. Toss in the chopped up scallion and shiitake mushrooms and sauté them for about 5 minutes
9. Toss in the Kimchi to the same pan and let the juices boil up for about 4-5 minutes
10. Toss in the pork and cook for a few minutes extra to make sure everything is finely done.

<u>Nutrition Values(Per Serving)</u>

- Protein: 27.3g
- Carbs: 9.5g
- Fats: 20g
- Calories: 334

Chapter 5: Desert Recipes

Creamy Pumpkin Fudge

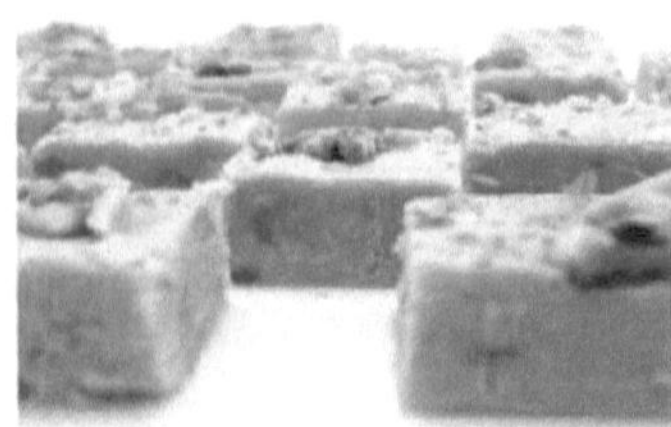

Serving: 25

Prep Time: 15 minutes

Cook Time: 120 minutes

Ingredients

- 1 and a ¾ cup of coconut butter
- 1 cup of pumpkin puree
- 1 teaspoon of ground cinnamon
- ¼ teaspoon of ground nutmeg
- 1 tablespoon of coconut oil

How To

1. Take an 8x8 inch square baking pan and line it with aluminum foil to start with

2. Take a spoon of scoop up the coconut butter into a heated pan and let the butter melt over low heat

3. Keep stirring it and remove the heat gently

4. Toss in the spices and pumpkin and keep stirring it until a grainy texture has formed

5. Pour in the coconut oil and keep stirring it vigorously to make sure that everything is combined nicely

6. Scoop up the mixture into the previously prepared baking pan and distribute evenly

7. Place a piece of wax paper over the top of the mixture and press on the upper side to make evenly straighten up the topside

8. Remove the wax paper and throw it away

9. Place the mixture into your fridge and let it cool for about 1-2 hours

10. Take it out and cut it into slices, then eat

<u>Nutrition Values(Per Serving)</u>

- Protein: 1.2g
- Carbs: 4.2g
- Fats: 10.7g
- Calories: 120

Soft Caprese Salad

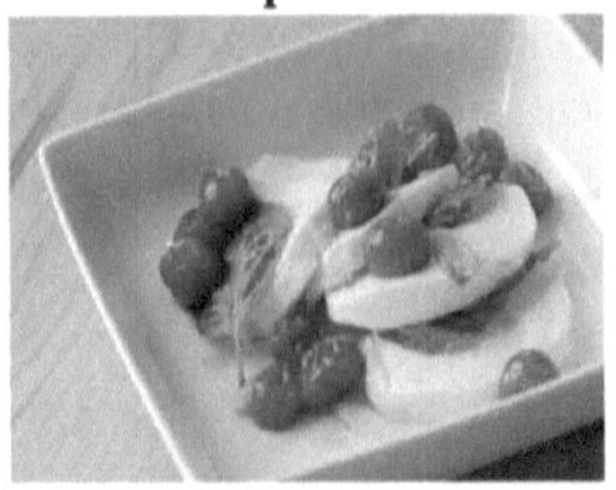

Serving: 2

Prep Time: 10 minutes

Cook Time: 0minutes

Ingredients

- 1 piece of Fresh Tomato
- 6 ounce of Fresh Mozzarella Cheese
- 1/3 a cup of chopped up Fresh Basil
- 3 tablespoon of Olive oil
- Freshly Cracked Black Pepper
- Salt

How To

1. Take a food processor and pulse up your freshly chopped up basil leaves with 2 tablespoons of Olive Oil and turn into a fine paste
2. Slice up your tomatoes into ¼ inch slices
3. Cut up your Mozzarella into 1-ounce slices
4. Assemble your Caprese salad by dish out layers of tomato, basil leaves and mozzarella
5. Season it up with some extra olive oil, pepper and salt as needed
6. Serve

Nutrition Values

- Protein: 15g
- Carbs: 3.5g
- Fats: 36g

- Calories: 405

Very Intense Sage And Cheddar Waffles

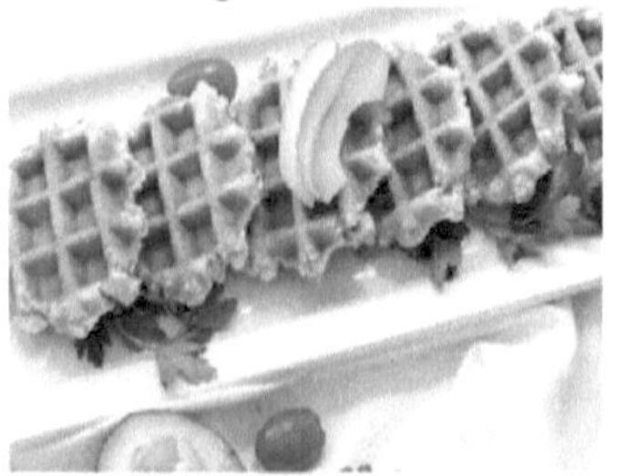

Serving: 12

Prep Time: 10 minutes

Cook Time: 10 minutes

Ingredients

- 1 and a 1/3 cup of sifted coconut flour
- 3 teaspoon of baking powder
- 1 teaspoon of dried ground sage
- ½ a teaspoon of salt
- ¼ a teaspoon of garlic powder
- 2 cups of canned coconut milk
- ½ a cup of water
- 2 pieces of egg
- 3 tablespoon of melted coconut oil
- 1 cup of shredded cheddar cheese

How To

1. The first step is to heat up your waffle iron and set it to moderate heat settings
2. Take a mixing bowl and toss in the baking powder, seasoning and flour and whisk them altogether nicely
3. Pour down all of the liquid ingredients and keep stirring until a nice batter forms
4. Toss in the cheese
5. Next up, open up your waffle iron and grease up the top and bottom sides

6. In about the waffle container, gently scoop of about 1/3 of the batter and pour it in the iron sections

7. Close down the Iron and let it cook until steam starts to rise from the top

8. Once done, open up your waffle iron and take out the waffles, to serve them hot.

9. Usually, you are going to need about 2 cycles of moderate heat to cook them properly

<u>Nutrition Values(Per Serving)</u>

- Protein: 6g
- Carbs: 3.81g
- Fats: 17g
- Calories: 213

•

Glamorous Apple Flatbread

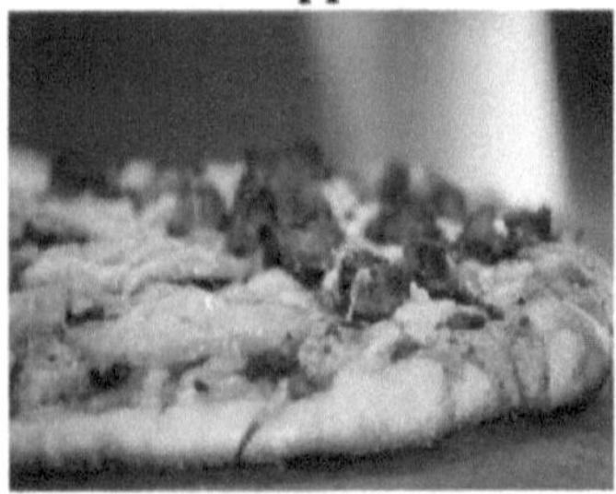

Serving: 8

Prep Time: 15 minutes

Cook Time: 15 minutes

Ingredients

Ingredients required for the crust

- 2 cups of grated partially skimmed mozzarella cheese
- ¾ cup of almond flour
- 2 tablespoon of sea salt
- 1/8 teaspoon of dried thyme

Ingredients required for the topping

- 2 cup of grated Mexican cheese
- ½ of a small onion sliced into thin portions
- ¼ of a medium sized apple. Seeded and cored with the skin intact
- 4 ounce of low carb ham sliced into chunks
- 1/8 teaspoon of dried thyme
- Salt as required
- Pepper as required

How To

1. The first step is to preheat your oven to a temperature of 425 degree Fahrenheit

2. Next, two about two pieces of parchment paper which should be about 2 inches large than a 12 inch pan pizza

3. Prepare a nice double boiler

4. Take a sauce pot and fill it up with just enough water and bring the water to simmer. Once brought to simmer, low down the heat

5. Take the mixing bowl prepared for the double boiler and toss in the cream cheese, mozzarella cheese, almond flour, salt and thyme

6. Gently place the bowl over the simmer pot and keep stirring it continuously while being careful of the steam

7. Once the cheese have melted down and ingredients are combined, pour down the mixture to one of the previously prepared parchment paper and knead it for a few minutes

8. Roll up the whole dough into a ball and place it on the center of the paper

9. Gently keep patting it until a nice circular shape has appeared

10. Cover it with the other parchment paper.

11. Take a rolling pin and keep rolling the dough until it has a nice 12-inch radius

12. Place the prepared dough on a pizza pan and take a fork to drill holes all over

13. Bake it for about 8 minutes

14. Once a golden texture has appeared, lower down the heat to 350 degrees Fahrenheit

15. Sprinkle about ¼ cup of the cheese

16. Finely place the sliced onion, apple and ham

17. Bake it again for 5-7 minutes until the cheese has melted and browned

18. Place it on a cooling rack and let it cool for about 3 minutes before cutting into 8 individual slices

<u>Nutrition Values(Per Serving)</u>

- Protein: 16g
- Carbs: 4g
- Fats: 20g
- Calories: 255

The Greatest McGriddle Casserole

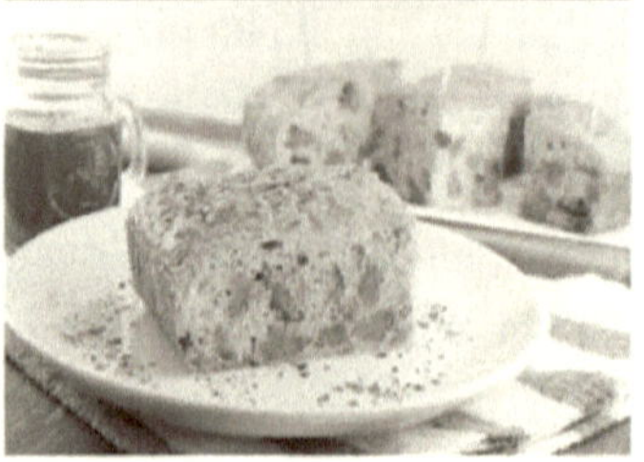

Serving: 8

Prep Time: 15 minutes

Cook Time: 40 minutes

Ingredients

- 1 cup of almond flour
- ¼ cup of Flaxseed Meal
- 1 pound of breakfast sausage
- 10 large pieces of eggs
- 4 ounce of cheddar cheese
- 6 tablespoon of Walden Farms Maple Syrup
- 4 tablespoon of Butter
- ½ a teaspoon of Onion Powder
- ½ a teaspoon of Garlic Powder
- ¼ teaspoon of Sage
- Salt as required
- Pepper as required

How To

1. Pre-heat your oven to a temperature of 350 degrees Fahrenheit
2. Take your pan and put on your stove over medium heat and toss in the breakfast sausage and break it up while cooking
3. Take a separate bowl and in that bowl, toss in all the dry ingredients and then toss in all of the wet ingredients
4. Toss in just 4 tablespoons of syrup and mix everything finely
5. Once the sausage are browned, pour in the mixture and mix again a little bit more

6. Prepare a 9x9 casserole dish using a parchment paper and pour in the casserole mixture in the dish
7. Use 2 tablespoons and drizzle them over the final mixture
8. Place it in the oven and let it bake for about 45-55 minutes
9. Remove it slowly lift It out, and serve

Nutrition Values(Per Serving)

- Protein: 22.6g
- Carbs: 2.9g
- Fats: 41g
- Calories: 481
- Fiber: 2.5g

Miniature Vanilla Cloud Muffins

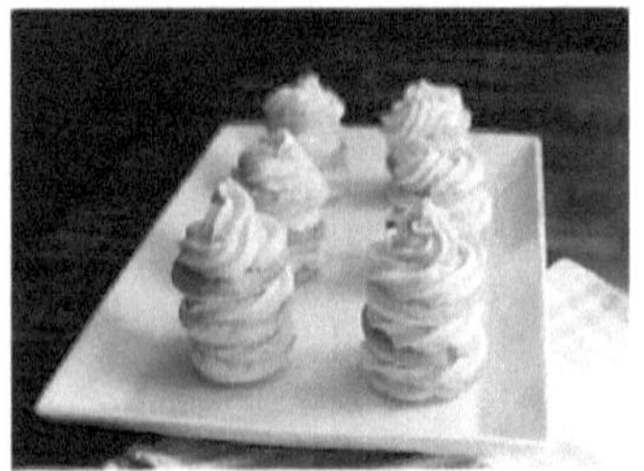

Serving: 8

Prep Time: 15 minutes

Cook Time: 40 minutes

Ingredients

For the cake

- 6 pieces of large separated large eggs
- 6 tablespoon of cream cheese at room temperature
- ½ a teaspoon of tartar cream
- 2 teaspoon of vanilla extract
- ¼ cup of granulated stevia

For the Frosting

- 16 ounce of softened cream cheese
- 2 tablespoon of butter
- 1/3 cup of granulated stevia
- 1 tablespoon of vanilla extract

How To

1. Pre-heat your oven to a temperature of 300 degrees Fahrenheit

2. Take about 2 muffin tins and grease them with spray oil

3. Take a medium sized bowl and toss in the cream cheese, sweetener, egg yolks, vanilla extract until a nice smooth consistency has been achieved

4. Take another bowl, and whip the tartar cream and egg whites using a mixer until a foam appears

5. Then, gently pour in the whites mixture to the yolk mixture

6. Scoop up about 2 tablespoons of the mixture into each of the muffin tins

7. Place it in the oven for 30-35 minutes until browned

8. Take them out and let it cool on a cooling rack

9. Take another bowl and mix in all the ingredients of the frosting and beat with a mixer

10. Move the frosting into a pastry bag and put a layer of frosting between on top a cake, and put another cake on top of the frosting. Make a total of three layers.

<u>Nutrition Values(Per Serving)</u>

- Protein: 10g
- Carbs: 5g
- Fats: 30g
- Calories: 347

Very Refreshing Lemon Popsicles

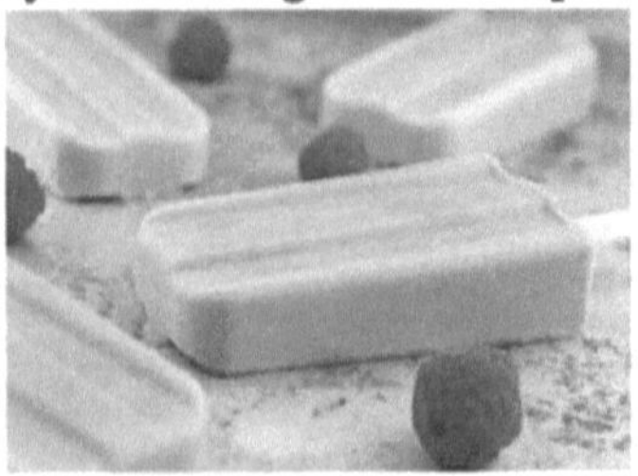

Serving: 6

Prep Time: 10 minutes

Cook Time: 120 minutes

Ingredients

- 100g of Raspberries
- Juice of ½ a lemon
- ¼ cup of coconut oil
- 1 cup of coconut milk
- ¼ cup of sour cream
- ¼ cup of heavy cream
- ½ a teaspoon of Guar Gum
- 20 drops of Liquid Stevia

How To

1. Take an immersion blender and toss in all of the ingredients and blend them altogether nicely

2. Once done, take them mixture through a mesh and strain the mixture, discarding all of the raspberry seeds

3. Pour in the mixture into a mold and keep the mold inside the fridge for 2 hours

4. Once done, pass the mold through hot water to dislodge the popsicles

Nutrition Values(Per Serving)

- Protein: 0.5g
- Carbs: 2g
- Fats: 16g

- Calories: 150

Generous Coconut Orange Creamsicles!

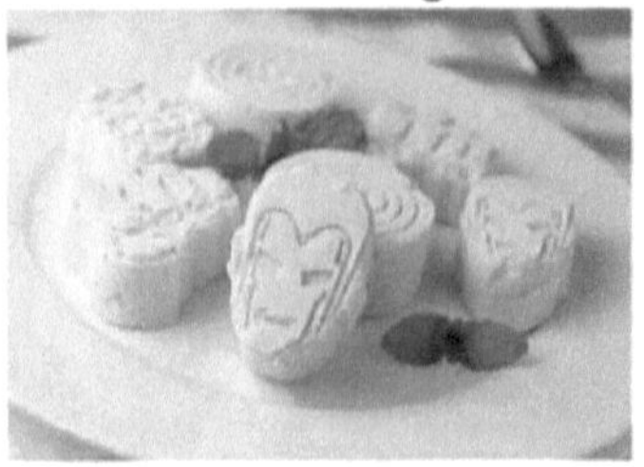

Serving: 10

Prep Time: 10 minutes

Cook Time: 180 minutes

Ingredients

- ½ a cup of coconut oil
- ½ a cup of heavy whipping cream
- 4 ounce of cream cheese
- 1 teaspoon of orange vanilla Mio
- 10 drops of liquid stevia

How To

1. Take an immersion blender and mix in all of the ingredients and blend them up

2. Take the mixture and pour it into the silicone tray and let it freeze for about 2-3 hours

3. Once it is hardened properly, finely remove the silicone tray and eat it up

Nutrition Values(Per Serving)

- Protein: 0.8g
- Carbs: 0.7g
- Fats: 20g
- Calories: 176

Conclusion

I would like to thank you for purchasing and downloading my book. I really do hope that you had a pleasant time with my book and enjoyed reading it.

I bid you farewell and hope that your Keto journey may turn out to be a huge success! I would feel that I have accomplished my mission even I had a tiny contribution to helping you achieve a healthy lifestyle

Stay healthy and stay safe.

www.ingramcontent.com/pod-product-compliance
Lightning Source LLC
Chambersburg PA
CBHW020739160726
47993CB00006B/2524